Santa C
School District
Special Education

W9-CRS-889

The Evolving Brain

Also by Tony Buzan

Speed Memory
Speed Reading
Use Your Head
Make the Most of Your Mind
Spore One

The Evolving Brain

Tony Buzan and Terence Dixon

HOLT, RINEHART & WINSTON
New York, Chicago, San Francisco, Dallas

Copyright 1978
ISBN: 0-03-044581-7   **Holt, Rinehart & Winston**

First published in the United States of America
by Holt, Rinehart & Winston
CBS Educational Publishing
A Division of CBS, Inc

Printed in Great Britain

Contents

CONTENTS

1 The Enchanted Loom

The human brain and its potential

The human brain is an enchanted loom where millions of flashing shuttles weave a dissolving pattern, always a meaningful pattern, though never an abiding one. It is as if the Milky Way entered upon some cosmic dance.

Sir Charles Sherrington

To compare the brain with a galaxy is in fact a modest analogy. Every intact person on our planet carries around his three-and-a-half-pound mass of tissue without giving much thought to it; but every normal brain is capable of making more patterned interconnections than there are atoms in the universe.

The brain is composed of about ten billion nerve cells and each one is capable of being involved in a vast series of complex connections thousands of times every second. At a mathematical level alone, the complexity is astounding. There are ten billion neurons in the brain and each one has a potential of connections of 10^{28}. In more comprehensible terms, it means that if the theoretical number of potential connections were to be written out, we would get a figure beginning with 1 and followed by about ten million kilometres of noughts.

All this is potential, of course, and, despite the manifold detailed discoveries of neurophysiology, many of which are dealt with in this book, it is the brain's potential which is most exciting. It is undisputed that we all underuse our brains—if we do not actually abuse them. This is hardly surprising. Few of us will ever see a human brain. Those who have do not describe it as a particularly remarkable sight. It is understandable that a concert pianist or a carpenter should value his hands above all, that a painter should

7

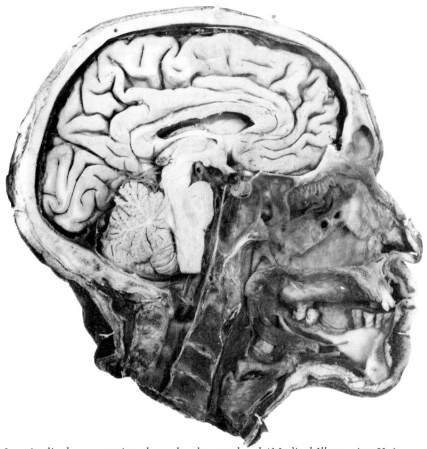

Longitudinal cross section through a human head (*Medical Illustration Unit, Royal College of Surgeons*)

cherish his eyes, that a runner should be most concerned about his legs. But hands are as useless without a brain as the piano itself without a player. The brain's potential has been largely under-estimated just because of its omnipresence. It is involved in all we do, in everything that happens to us, and so we note that which is different in each experience, overlooking perhaps that without which nothing is possible for us.

We have been too much concerned with differential rather than potential in another, more important, sense. Since we have known that such things as brains existed we have devoted most of our efforts

8

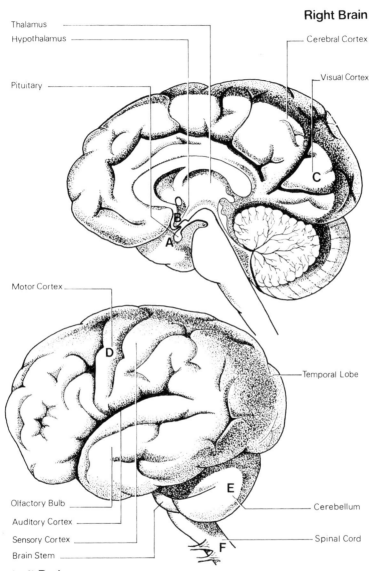

Right Brain

Thalamus

Hypothalamus

Cerebral Cortex

Visual Cortex

Pituitary

C

Motor Cortex

D

Temporal Lobe

Olfactory Bulb

E

Auditory Cortex

Cerebellum

Sensory Cortex

Spinal Cord

Brain Stem

F

Left Brain
Cross section of the two sides of the brain: A, Pituitary (controls water balance and all the hormones); B, Hypothalamus (controls primitive emotions and appetites); C, Visual Cortex (receives and analyses visual input); D, Motor Cortex (initiates voluntary movement); E, Cerebellum (harmonises balance and voluntary muscular movement); F, Spinal Cord (transmits and relays messages through the rest of the spinal column)

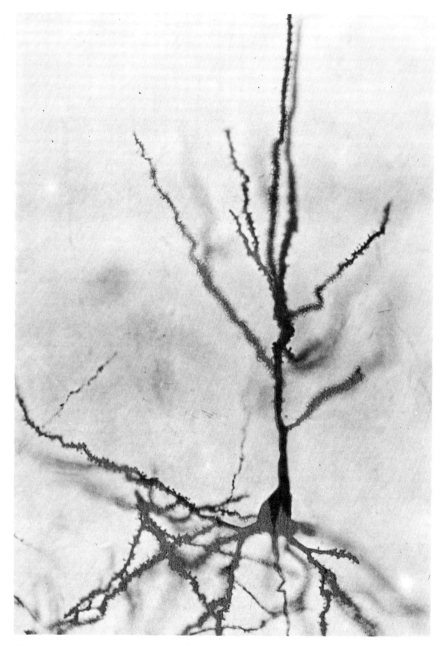

A neuron from a cat's cortex, Golgi–Cox stain (*A. J. Aldrich*)

not to improving them but to devising systems to demonstrate the differences between them. This applies not only in education, where pass or fail is the ultimate criterion, but in every aspect of our lives. We are American or Chinese, scholar or peasant, artist or scientist. These distinctions exist, of course, and it would be foolish to dismiss them completely. But the inherent ability of each brain in its own right is important too. In every head is a formidable powerhouse, a compact, efficient organ whose capacity seems to expand further towards infinity the more we learn of it.

John Rader Platt expressed this view:

> If this property of complexity could somehow be transformed into visible brightness so that it would stand forth more clearly to our senses, the biological world would become a walking field of light compared to the physical world. The sun with its great eruptions would fade to a pale simplicity compared to a rose bush, an earthworm would be a beacon, a dog would be a city of light, and human beings would stand out like blazing suns of complexity, flashing bursts of meaning to each other through the dull night of the physical world between. We would hurt each other's eyes. Look at the haloed heads of your rare and complex companions. Is it not so?

The basis of this 'property of complexity' is the nerve cell—the neuron. Even those which are microscopically small are in themselves remarkably complex. Neurons differ from most other cells in that they are a more complicated shape and have many branching prolongations which can connect with each other to transmit nerve impulses. Throughout the nervous system the neurons vary tremendously in size. Some, running from the toes or the fingers into the spinal cord, can be as much as a metre in length. Others, in the cerebral cortex for example, are more than a thousand times smaller.

Everything we do, from moving a muscle to thinking great thoughts, involves intricate neuronal functioning. Whatever the activity, however, the process is similar and is founded on the excitation of the neuron. The process consists of electro-chemical signals being passed from one neuron to another: not just singly or slowly but in rapid, multiple waves of communication. Each neuron has a main body which contains specific chemical and genetic

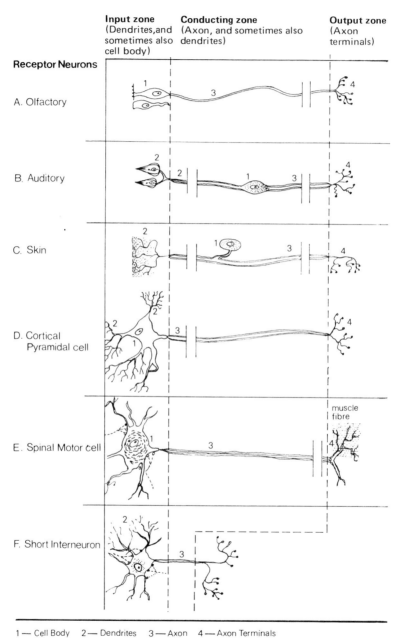

Receptor neurons, showing some of the variations in neurone shape according to function

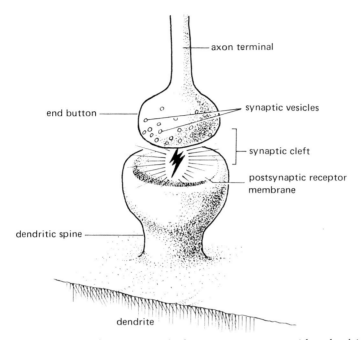

An artist's impression of a synapse which connects an axon with a dendrite

information and an axon which conducts the vital nerve impulses. It will also have a variable number of branching dendrites. These are the receivers of the impulses or information, either directly from a sense organ or, more commonly, from other neurons in the tapestry of connections.

The precise location of the transmission of the impulse from one neuron to another is the synapse where the information 'flows' across a microscopic gap not unlike the spark plug gap or the distributor points in the internal combustion engine. The physics and chemistry of this process are immensely intricate. In the synapse chemical substances are released which enable the electrical impulses to be transmitted and the synapse has a threshold which affects how readily the impulse is accepted. In familiar or reflex activity the threshold is lower so that the circuit operates more readily. A higher threshold means that the signal is more difficult to transmit.

An impulse from a single neuron causes activation in the synapses it forms with others and even the simplest mental or physical process

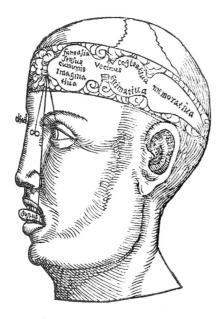

A medieval illustration of the three 'cerebral ventricles' where the mental faculties were supposed to reside (*Ronan Picture Library & E. P. Goldschmidt & Co Ltd*)

involves certainly hundreds of neurons receiving and transmitting impulses in complex cascading waves of communication and co-operation. A hundred thousand neuronal 'messages' a second is commonplace.

Everything we do and experience, therefore, involves this intricate bio-electrical process — from playing tennis to paying the bills. This is not as perplexing as it might seem. We know that the eyes do not in themselves see: they are merely lenses. The ears do not in themselves hear: they are, so to speak, microphones. When we watch a cricket match on television we do not see the players themselves but electronic representations of them on the picture tube. What is between the cat you see in the flesh and your brain's image of the cat is a series of neurophysiological processes, just as there is a series of electronic processes between the actual cricket match and the image you see on television.

Obviously the synaptic threshold is of great importance in terms of efficient functioning. We know, for example, that in emergency situations extra adrenalin is generated in our bloodstream. This lowers our synaptic threshold, stimulates our reactions and we are able to act faster and—theoretically—more effectively. A significant

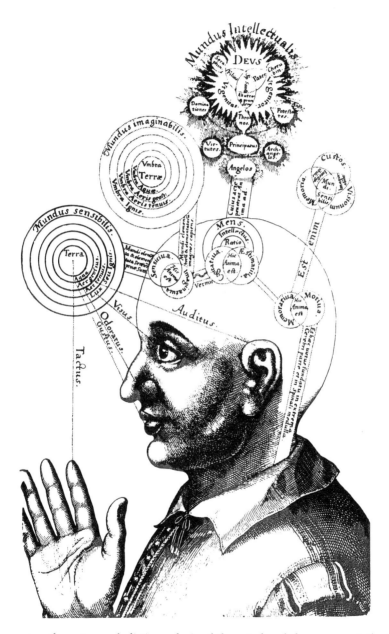

A seventeenth-century cabalistic analysis of the mind and the senses, attributing different functions to different regions of the brain (*Ronan Picture Library & E. P. Goldschmidt & Co Ltd*)

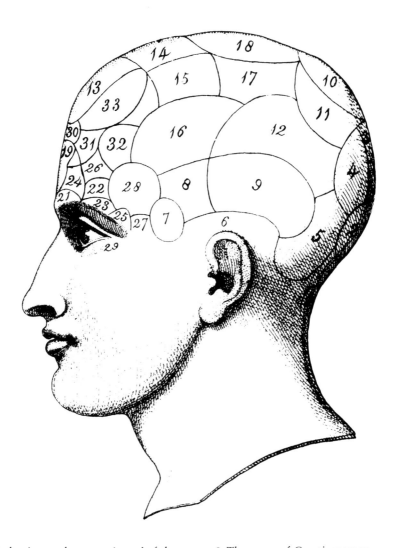

Early nineteenth-century 'maps' of the brain produced by Gall and Spurzheim based on phrenology (*Ronan Picture Library & E. P. Goldschmidt & Co Ltd*)

1 The organ of Amativeness
2 The organ of Philoprogenativeness
3 The organ of Inhabitiveness
4 The organ of Adhesiveness
5 The organ of Combativeness
6 The organ of Destructiveness
7 The organ of Constructiveness
8 The organ of Covetiveness or Acquisitiveness
9 The organ of Secretiveness
10 Self-Love or Self-Esteem
11 Love of Approbation
12 Organ of Cautiousness
13 Organ of Benevolence
14 The organ of Veneration, or of Theosophy
15 The organ of Hope
16 Ideality, or the Poetical Disposition

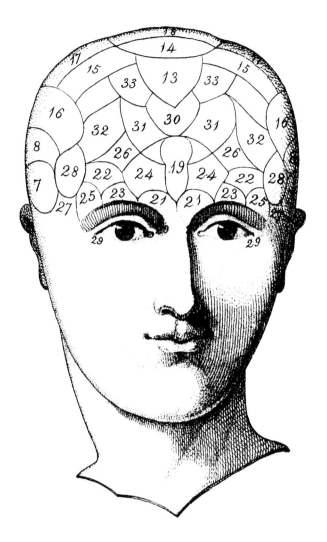

17 The organ of Righteousness, or
   Conscientiousness
18 Determinateness
19 Individuality
20 The organ of Form
21 The organ of Size
22 The organ of Weight
23 The organ of Colour
24 The organ of Space
25 The organ of Order
26 The organ of Time

27 The organ of Number
28 The organ of Tune
29 The organ of Language
30 The organ of Comparison
31 The organ of Causality
32 The organ of Wit
33 The organ of Imitation

Key to numbers on illustrations of
phrenology from *Encyclopaedia
Londinensis*, Vol. xx, London, 1825

amount of modern psychiatric treatment is based on chemical interference at this level. It is argued that some mental disorders are caused by inefficient synapses with weak chemical transmitters which produce the neurological equivalent of a poor sparking plug. In some cases patients are treated with the introduction of extra doses of synapse transmitter chemicals, for example noradrenalin. This does appear to alleviate the symptoms of lethargy and depression. Conversely, a tranquilizing effect is obtained by using chlorpromazine which blocks the release of noradrenalin at the synapse. All this is borne out by more ancient everyday experience. We know that a cup of strong coffee 'bucks us up', for example, or that a cigarette (whatever else it does) 'calms our nerves'. Caffeine, the drug contained in coffee, does in fact lower the synaptic threshold so that activity is artificially made that much easier. The nicotine in tobacco, on the other hand, raises thresholds, effectively deadens reactions, and thus has an apparent calming effect.

More will be said of the brain's chemistry later, but it is useful first to look more closely at the anatomy of the brain. Although the 'map' of the brain is by no means complete—about two-thirds of its volume still defies 'job description'—it does divide into four main sections. Each section has specific but intricately connected, complementary and even overlapping functions.

The famous grey matter itself—that part which would be immediately visible if one looked at a removed brain—is the cerebral cortex, also known as the cerebrum or the cerebral hemispheres. There are in fact two symmetrical hemispheres, closely connected but visibly distinct. It is of interest, though so far inexplicable, that the left hemisphere appears to regulate functions involving the right side of the body and vice versa. Chapter 6 contains much more discussion of the discoveries and theories concerning the two hemispheres.

Like most of the brain, the cerebral cortex is extensively fissured and folded. Even in the simplest anatomical sense there is more to it than meets the eye. If opened out, the cortex of the average adult would measure more than two square feet. The size of the cortex, in relation to the rest of the brain, is in proportion to the level of its owner on the evolutionary tree. Man has the largest, the primates rather less, smaller mammals still less, and many creatures—birds

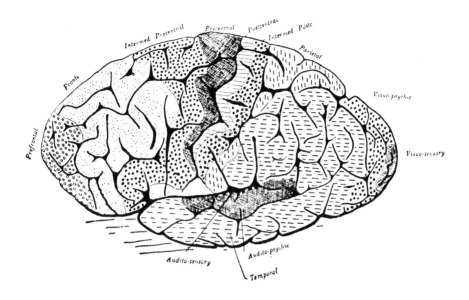

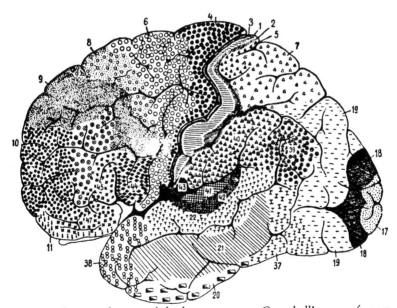

Two cytoarchitectural maps of the human cortex. Campbell's map of 1905 (above) the prototype of all subsequent charts of the human brain and Brodmann's map of 1909 (below) giving his numerical designation of principal areas (*Anne Horton*)

for example—have none at all. Not surprisingly, therefore, the cerebral cortex is the seat of such so-called higher functions in Man as thought and intelligence, as well as the centre of a great deal of vital neuronal activity concerning, for example, speech and sight.

The second section is often referred to as the 'old brain'—'old' in the evolutionary sense. This is the area in the middle of the brain, covered by the cortex, and also known as the limbic system. The control of instinctive and, to some extent, emotional behaviour is located here. A particular part of the system, the hypothalamus, is also concerned with the regulation of the autonomic nervous system which controls the inner workings of the body—blood pressure, heart rate, digestion and so on. Recently, it has been shown that these autonomic responses are by no means as automatic as had been supposed (see particularly Chapter 6). This is not as surprising as it might appear, since it has long been known that 'thoughts' in the cerebral cortex can effect autonomic responses supervised by the old brain; hence stomach ulcers apparently caused by worry and high blood pressure seeming to result from stress.

The cerebellum, the third main section, lies to the rear of the brain. This is the master control of motor activity, the body's physical movement. It is the neuronal activity in the cerebellum which enables the precise co-ordination of eye and limb and movement which we all take for granted. Although it is capable of being controlled by what might be called motivation in the cerebral cortex, the cerebellum is also quite capable of, so to speak, independent activity. For example, while you are driving your car, your cerebral cortex may 'decide' that it is time to switch the lights on. A message is flashed to the cerebellum, the muscles are co-ordinated and a small switch on a dark dashboard is located and operated. You may then continue to contemplate the personal problem that has occupied you and mean-while the cerebellum continues to enable all the muscular and related activities involved in driving the car without requiring any very intense conscious (cerebral) thought.

Of course the brain as a whole is operating as long as the body is functioning normally and the above actions would also involve the specific activity regulated by the remaining main section of the brain, the brain stem. This is the stalk-like lower part of the brain which is anatomically the continuation, or culmination, of the spinal column.

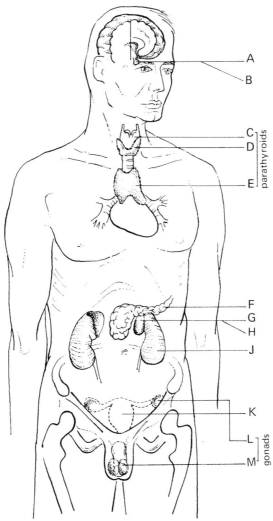

The brain controls the glandular system, which in its turn controls the physical development of the body and many of its functions: A, anterior pituitary (the 'master gland'; its hormones influence secretions of the thyroid, pancreas, adrenal cortex, and gonads. Also secretes growth hormones); B, posterior pituitary (water metabolism, salt metabolism, etc); C, thyroid cartilage; D, thyroid (metabolic rate); E, thymus (lymph system, immune reactions); F, Pancreas (insulin, controls sugar metabolism); G, adrenal cortex – outer bark (controls salt and carbohydrate metabolism; controls inflammatory reactions); H, adrenal medulla – inner core (active in emotional arousal and sleep through its hormones ephinephrine and norepinephrine); J, kidney; K, uterus L, ovary and M, testis (produce hormones that affect bodily development and that maintain reproductive organs in adults)

It is from here that certain basic organic functions such as breathing are supervised. It also appears that the stem houses some of the brain's ability to select, from an almost infinite amount of incoming data, that which is relevant to its basic interest or immediate purpose. It seems that the brain stem contains, for example, the mechanism which enables a mother to sleep through persistent heavy traffic but awaken at her baby's slightest whimper.

It is important to remember, however, that for all its specificity and localised functions, the brain is fundamentally and primarily an integrated organ. The distinguished Russian neuropsychologist, Professor Luria, argues that the brain must be considered to operate as a *function system* (see Chapter 4). This means that the brain is not just a conglomerate of interconnected working parts but an infinitely more self-regulating system. In other words, the brain is not a system of isolated functions, but a system designed to fulfil an *overall* function. What is more, there is encouraging evidence from Luria himself that, in consequence, other parts of the brain can be trained to take over the work of damaged areas.

An extraordinary example of how the undamaged part of a brain can somehow compensate is to be found in the case of a Portuguese woman named Maria. At the age of five she was half-paralyzed and the sight of her left eye was severely affected by damage to the right-hand side of her brain. Subsequently, she suffered acute epileptic seizures until, by the time she was twenty, she was frequently uncontrollable. In desperation, her doctors removed her entire right hemisphere. The transformation was as rapid and remarkable as it is inexplicable. Within a month she was able to walk and now, at the age of thirty-four, she does housework and cares for a young child. She has no need of treatment.

Since the righthand side of the brain controls, for the most part, the lefthand side of the body, Maria's recovery is theoretically impossible. And yet the paralysis of the lefthand side of her body is cured. The leftside functions, though weaker than the right, are within a normal range. Her left eye is not quite blind and the right eye's visual field has considerably expanded to compensate. She has reasonable hearing in her left ear.

Cases like Maria's are so exceptional that they provide dangerous springboards for wide generalisation. It is clear, however, that

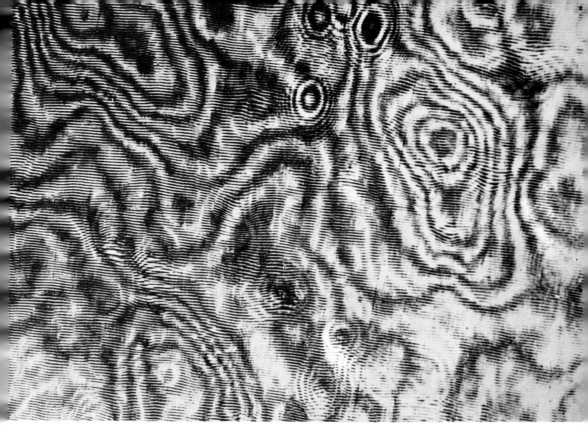

The surface of a holographic plate in white light (*Michael Wenyon*)

although the study of specificity in the brain is useful for analysis and diagnosis, there is a great deal to be said for general research which concentrates on the brain as a holistic function system.

Attempts to locate the specific part of the brain where, for example, the apparently uniquely human quality of 'consciousness of consciousness' resided came to nothing. Similar difficulties were encountered in attempting to solve some of the complex problems of how memory works. It became clear, in fact, that such elusive phenomena were in some way distributed throughout the brain as a whole. It is difficult to visualise this complexity, but holographic photography gives us some idea of the process. The principle is esoteric, but in practice the system is as follows: an object is photographed using a technique involving a laser beam and recorded on a solid plate which can only reveal its image once again using laser light. The interesting point is that if the photographic plate thus produced is shattered it is possible to reproduce an image of the whole picture from just one tiny piece. The dramatic analogy

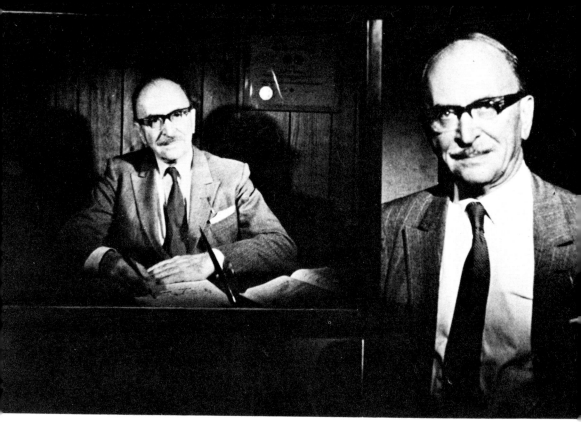

Dennis Gabor, the inventor, beside a holographic portrait of himself (R. Rhinehart, Macdonnell–Douglas Corporation)

between the hologram and the brain is that, just as the complete photographic information is dispersed through every fragment of the plate, so the basis of certain neurological functions may be distributed throughout the entire brain.

So far all this is what researchers call a 'model'. The research is incomplete and to some extent inconclusive. We do not yet know the details of the process in terms of the brain. What is clear, however, is that the power of the brain is greater and more complex than the sum of its parts and specific functions. Although it is able to do countless things simultaneously, the brain as a whole seems to be an essentially self-regulating system with, so to speak, an overall plan— the survival and success of the organism.

So far we have considered that which is common to all those who have a human brain. But we are all as different neurologically as we are physically. Each brain is unique, and it regulates an individual's character and personality as specifically as it enables different physical movements or organic functions. It does so because the nervous system is closely integrated with the endocrine glands, of which the main one—the pituitary—is joined to the base of the brain itself. These glands secrete hormones which carry chemical messages throughout the bloodstream to produce specific efforts in what are called the target organs.

The secretion of some hormones is directly controlled by neurons and there are close anatomical links between the brain itself and the endocrine glands. Axons from the hypothalamus, for example, synapse in the pituitary. Another electro-chemical integration may be observed in the fact that the hormone noradrenalin which, as we have seen, is employed by the nervous system as a synaptic transmitter, is closely related to adrenalin which is secreted into the bloodstream by the adrenal glands.

The dominant endocrine gland is the pituitary which is substantially involved in the regulation of other glands and the production of their hormones.

Let us take an example of this neurophysiological system in action. I see a man about to attack my wife. I consciously realise the danger (in my cerebral cortex); the alarm is immediately sent to the hypothalamus which stimulates (via the pituitary) the adrenal glands. As a result of this stimulation, the hormonal messages cause my heart to pump more blood to the muscles, my blood sugar increases to feed muscle action, I breathe more deeply to increase the oxygen content of the bloodstream. In short, my body is prepared for vigorous action.

Needless to say, the physical aspects are only part of such an experience. If such an event took place, one would be aware of what can only be called emotional response as well. This combination of mental and physical—of neuronal and hormonal—responses accounts for a great deal of what we describe as abstract 'feelings'. Fear, anger, sexuality, even jealousy and competition are all in part as attributable to brain/gland interaction as hunger and thirst.

Some contemporary research even indicates that our perception of pain may, in some measure, be a function of the chemistry of the brain. It has been observed for some time that morphine and other pain-killing opiates work, like the brain's own chemicals, by attaching themselves to those neurons that influence the pain threshold. Now researchers as far apart as China and Scotland have found that the brain can in fact manufacture its own pain-killing 'drugs' which, not surprisingly, work in the same way as morphine, etc.

Chinese scientists recently reported that acupuncture, when used as an anaesthetic, caused the brain of a rabbit to produce analgesic chemicals known as enkaphalins. In his recent Reith Lecture, Dr Colin Blakemore, the Cambridge neurologist, commented: 'Morphine and the related compound, heroin, are dangerously addictive drugs and their unsupervised possession is illegal; yet we all carry within our heads a "natural opiate" that our brains use to regulate this most fundamental aspect of our consciousness — the perception of pain.'

This connection between morphine and the so-called 'natural opiate' was soon perceived to be of practical as well as theoretical interest. It was observed that the introduction of doses of an enkaphalin known as beta-endorphin created in rats a physical rigidity that closely resembled catatonic schizophrenia in humans. Since a drug called nalaxone is used to counteract the effects of morphine, it was clearly theoretically possible that it could be used to counteract the effects of morphine's 'natural' counterpart. Sure enough, in an experiment at the Salk Institute in California, an injection of nalaxone completely cured the 'catatonia' induced in rats by beta-endorphin. To complete the connection, experiments using nalaxone with schizophrenic patients at the University of Uppsala in Sweden have produced encouraging results.

Mention has already been made of the effects of drugs on 'mental processes'. There is little doubt that a clearer and profounder understanding of the subtleties and complexities of the brain's chemistry will result in more helpful treatment for what are currently thought of as psychological—as opposed to physiological—disorders.

It is certainly clear that even with the evidence now available there is considerable danger in the continuing use of such blunt and irrevocable treatments as brain surgery and electro-convulsive-therapy.

But we are not all just helpless receptacles of the effects of our own brain chemistry. Nor is it true that the use of drugs is the only way to modify our response. Once again, let us consider noradrenalin. Research has shown that the production of this vital hormone works on the syndrome principle. To put it simply, the more your brain produces, the more it can make, and vice versa. If someone on the downward spiral—making less and less—gets into a clinical condition, the chemical can be artificially introduced. And, as has already been said, symptoms of depression and lethargy can be relieved. But self-help is possible without drugs. We all experience days when 'nothing goes right', when family or friends appear to have 'got out of the wrong side of the bed' and continue the day with increasing depression. These are simply everyday descriptions of the reducing noradrenalin production syndrome. The cure is simply to reverse the spiral. If your day starts badly, it might well—all things being equal—get worse. We all know that sudden good news or some unexpected pleasantness can cheer us up and lift depression—raise noradrenalin production. If that does not happen, the answer is deliberately to generate a series of successes, however small, to accelerate secretion of the vital hormone. When you get to work, do something that you had been putting off. If you are at home, clean out a cupboard you had been meaning to for weeks. Follow that with any other tasks which you can easily but successfully do and press on upwards. It works. It is common sense. Your brain 'knows' it already.

The fact that body chemistry regulates certain emotional states does not imply that we are helpless, circumscribed hominoids any more than the fact of genetic inheritance reduces us as individuals. All human beings share a substantial common ground of emotions. At different times, in various ways, under certain circumstances, we all experience anxiety, reassurance, emotional pain and pleasure. The fact that, as and when these states of mind and body exist, we can to some extent 'explain' them is not to diminish our own uniqueness. I may be enraged by something which makes you laugh and another cry. In fact, the more we are able to identify the basis of states of 'mind' in general, the more remarkable it is that the human unit remains so infinite in its variety.

Having examined some of the factors affecting the internal workings of the brain, it is now appropriate to consider some work being done on the inter-relationship between the brain and the external world.

For many years, sociologists have made the point that our environment has a considerable effect on us—slums breed delinquency and so on. In parallel with this, neurological research has demonstrated that the environment can create measurable changes in the brain

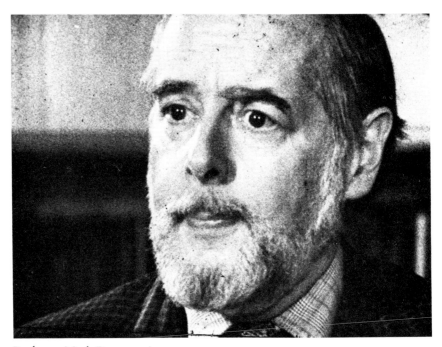

Professor Mark Rosenzweig

itself. At the moment most of this work is being done on the brains of rats, and while direct comparison with humans is tentative, certain correlations are plausible. At Berkeley University in California, Professor Mark Rosenzweig has been conducting experiments in controlled environments which provide rats with different degrees of stimulation. A number of rats is divided into two groups. The first is kept in what Rosenzweig describes as 'baseline conditions' for laboratory animals—three to a cage with adequate provision of food, drink and attention. The others are kept in larger groups of a dozen or so in much bigger cages which are filled with interesting objects for the animals to climb on, smell, make sounds with, generally explore and play among. The objects are rearranged each day to provide a continuously changing and stimulating environment.

Rosenzweig has demonstrated that the differences between the two groups of rats, even after quite a short time, is remarkable. Those animals from the larger cages—the enriched environment— manifest considerable changes, chemical and anatomical, in their brains. They have heavier and thicker cerebral cortices, larger neuronal cell bodies and neuronal nuclei. They were also found to have more ribonucleic acid (RNA) per cell. RNA controls and directs the formation of protein in cells, and since protein synthesis is responsible for the growth of cells and the production of chemical transmitters at the synapse, Rosenzweig argues that the enriched environment 'means that the cells become more active'. These rats were also found to be friendlier and easier to handle.

In addition, independent tests on Rosenzweig's rats found an increase in the number of dendritic spines in the animals from the enriched environment. Other researches at the University of Illinois have found that these animals produced a denser, more intricate pattern of neuronal branching. And so, when the animals have a sufficiently rich environment, the neurons are more active, are making more branches to connect with each other, and are making better connections.

Another optimistic discovery of Rosenzweig's—and one he is more confident about relating to human beings—concerns the continuing plasticity or flexibility of the brain. He has found that even when his laboratory rats are quite old, three weeks' exposure to the enriched environment enables them to catch up with their litter-mates who have been in it since birth. Rosenzweig considers this to be 'a very hopeful thing'. As he says:

> When I have spoken about continuing plasticity in the brain, I have found some people very reluctant to accept the results— people who supposed that human intelligence and personality are very well set by experiences of just the first few years of life. But I think the trend is changing, and I now find among developmental psychologists much more interest in the continuing capacity to learn and change. It is certainly true of our rats, and I think it is true of people, that not all our lives are determined by the first three years, but that we have a great deal of opportunity to grow and develop after that.

This work has obvious significance in terms not only of the way we think about early development, but also of ageing. Rosenzweig also says:

> The decline of mental ability with age does not seem to be

inevitable. My hope is that it will be found that many people can be helped to continue an active mental life well into advanced age. It may well be that sufficient complexity of stimulation and experience will aid that. Certainly people never did evolve for inactivity.

A perennial problem is posed by the question: where does brain stop and mind start? Brain, it can be argued, is an organic, dissectable object and not sufficient to explain certain specifically human faculties. How, for example, can the appreciation of beauty or the love of God be a sequence of neuronal functions, however complex? This vexed problem is probably as old as Man's self-consciousness, and even though it may now be termed mind/brain dualism as distinct from what used to be called mind/body dualism, we are not much nearer a solution.

One approach to the mystery of metaphysical experience is to deny its existence at all. This argument is that abstract thought, aesthetic conceptions and so on are simply misleading bits of linguistics. Beauty, for example, is something which cannot be measured, scientifically analysed, or reproduced at will under laboratory conditions and is therefore, in a literal sense, in the eye (or rather the brain) of the beholder. According to this line of argument, beauty exists only in the language describing it and not in fact. The same applies to other mental states such as religious experience, some forms of altruism and so forth. In this scheme of things, morality becomes pragmatic politics, aesthetics becomes the physiology of perception, free will becomes determinism and psychology behaviourism.

In the behaviourist field, the seminal experimental work was done by Ivan Pavlov, of whom more in Chapter 4. His work on the conditioned reflex has been as influential in experimental psychology as Freud's theories have been in psychiatry. The ultimate argument of Pavlov's work is that the living organism must, in the last resort, be presumed to be of the same character as an automatic machine. It will, that is to say, only 'behave' in so far as it is caused to do so by a specific stimulus. The behaviourists, therefore, describe all behaviour in terms of responses to stimuli. The word stimulus is used in the widest sense to denote any change in the environment or physical condition of the organism. To prevent a bird from building its nest or an animal from feeding or mating, is to expose it to a stimulus. Similarly, the word 'response' is used in a wide sense to cover any form of behaviour from going to sleep, to addressing meetings, to having babies. The main purpose of this type of psychology is to be able to assign the cause of a particular aspect of behaviour by identifying the stimulus which produced it. The most influential behaviourist of our time is probably the American, B. F. Skinner. In his recent book, Skinner concludes that: 'A scientific analysis of behaviour must, I believe, assume that a person's behaviour is controlled by his genetic and environmental history rather than by the person himself as an initiating creative agent.' Whatever view one takes of this rather finite conclusion, it is impossible to ignore the substantial contribution Pavlov, Skinner and like-minded people have made to the study of the influence of the environment on the brain and behaviour. But the case against the behaviourist view has been well argued. For example, Robert Ornstein says in a recent book:

There was here an almost fatal confusion of 'behaviourism as a useful tool' with 'behaviourism as the total extent of knowledge'. 'Objective' factual knowledge was emphasised to the exclusion of any question not subject to a verbal, logical answer. The *reductio ad absurdum* of this position was that the Logical Positivists maintained that any question not amenable to a perfectly logical answer should not even be asked . . .
In psychology of late, the limitations of the successful behaviouristic paradigm have proven to outweigh the advances. To give one example, until recently psychologists have tended to ignore some evidence (from sources as diverse as Yoga and animal experiments) that man is capable of a high degree of self-mastery of his internal physiology . . .
In performing research, we are often unaware of the full effect of our tools, be they physical instruments or doctrines such as behaviourism. We often imagine that tools, like sensory organs, serve exclusively to extend awareness, but in fact we are wrong. Both serve to limit as well as extend.
Abraham Maslow, commenting on the effects of a strict behaviourism in psychology, said: 'If the only tool you have is a hammer, you tend to treat everything as if it were a nail'. A

corrective needs to be applied, one which can open up the scope of psychological inquiry to the relevant questions once again.

This fundamental controversy no doubt will continue to rage, from the pulpit to the classroom, into the foreseeable future. But, as A. N. Whithead said: 'A clash of doctrines is not a disaster—it is an opportunity'. Something of what is being made of this opportunity will be seen later in this book. Of particular interest in this context is the use of behaviourist-type laboratory experiments to demonstrate non-behaviourist theorist theories (see particularly chapters 4 and 6). It is sufficient to say here that the atmosphere in most areas of brain research at the moment is one of optimism and the expansion of possibilities. It is almost as if the age-old question 'are we really machines?' is being left in suspended animation in some academic corner while the astounding riches of the brain's ability are being pursued with conspicuous enthusiasm.

Our brains are, almost literally, everything. We can give more to them and in turn, and in addition, they can give to us. The brain is our secret, silent weapon. If we can just begin to use more of its power, we will indeed see a light that will hurt, but astonish, our eyes. To again quote John Rader Platt:

> Many of our most sensitive spirits today still see man as the anti-hero; the helpless victim of weapons and wars, of governments and mechanisms and soul-destroying organisations and computers — as indeed he is. But in the midst of this man-made and inhuman entropy, like a fourth law of man, there grows up, even in the laboratories, a realisation that man is also mysterious and elusive, self-determining and perpetual. A lighthouse of complexity and the organising child of the universe. One equipped and provided for to stand and choose and act and control and be.

2 An Afternoon at a London School

A practical demonstration of brain power

This chapter concerns a class of ten-year-olds in Poplar in the East End of London. It is about an experiment to demonstrate the application of brain research to teaching. This was not another attempt to impose a new technique which would sweep away all the others, but an opportunity for the children to realize their own almost unlimited possibilities. The children were generally considered to be 'non-academic material', many of them were hardly literate, even at this fairly advanced stage of their education.

The exercise lasted three hours and was conducted by Tony Buzan.

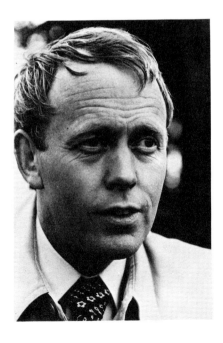

Tony Buzan

E.B.—C

To begin with, he asked the children to spend half an hour preparing a talk to give to the class. They were given a completely free choice of materials with which to prepare. A wide variety was available—ordinary pens, lined paper, blank paper of all sizes, felt-tipped pens of many colours and sizes. Each child took a generous selection of materials but at first used only the conventional pen or pencil and the lined paper.

During the half-hour period those children who were writing were unable, on average, to complete more than half a page; many of them were unable or unwilling even to start. Some did not use words at all and produced only a small drawing. Throughout the exercise they showed signs of restlessness, nervousness, discouragement and boredom. Many of them continually asked when the exercise would be over. The talks themselves were as dull as might be imagined. They were extremely brief and delivered with considerable reluctance. They ranged from a cursory reading of a few lines of written text to an almost subliminal 'I've done a picture of a motor'.

Buzan then began to persuade the children that they were in fact rather brighter than they thought. When the class was asked how many of them 'knew a lot' there was no response. Five minutes was then spent with the children raising their hands if they knew any of the following:

star	soil	publicity
house	eye	rubbish
plane	dog	knowledge
leather	happy	employment
sky	brain	anxious
tree	jungle	difficult
flower	music	custard
building	childhood	planets
glass	leopard	danger
watch	politician	possibility . . .
pencil	eagle	
river	typewriter	

After five minutes it was a considerable list. Every child, needless to say, scored 100%.

For the next ten minutes the children worked in pairs doing much the same exercise. They took it in turns to say words to each other and list how many they did not know. When this was completed—after fifteen minutes and the exchange of perhaps thousands of words—everyone still had a score of 100%. The class was then asked again how many 'knew a lot' and the response was considerably different. (The class in fact took upon themselves the role of knowledge missionaries and spent their next playtime proving to their friends in other classes that they were brighter than they thought too.)

The next stage was to demonstrate the uses to which this vast pool of word knowledge could be put. The idea of the multi-ordinate nature of words was introduced. It was explained to the children that each word has 'many hooks', that words have many connections which build up and up to form ideas, sentences, books, libraries! The example of a burr plant was used and the children were shown that each word has many more hooks than has a burr. It was emphasised that each mind would have different hooks for different words: that there were no 'right' or 'wrong' connections.

The children were then asked to write the word 'fish' in the middle of a blank page and to put their own hooks around it. They were encouraged to put any words that came into their minds, not just those that they thought were 'right'. It was also pointed out to them that they were generating their own hooks and not anyone else's and that, therefore, cheating would do them no good. It would simply prevent them from knowing what words their minds did connect with the starting word. The result was that the children virtually ignored each other and during the ten minutes available for the exercise each child managed at least fifteen associations of his own.

They were then shown that they could use the multi-hooked nature of words to overcome their fear of formal sentences and grammar. It was demonstrated, via two exercises, that their brains did not primarily use sentences and lines. In the first exercise the children were asked to write down ten sentences of ten words or more that they remembered from any source. After ten minutes no child had more than two sentences. This result was discussed and the children concluded that they did not in fact remember 'in sentences', but rather by important words, special images.

In the next exercise they were asked to 'look' at the way they thought. Each child sat for a few moments thinking and observing

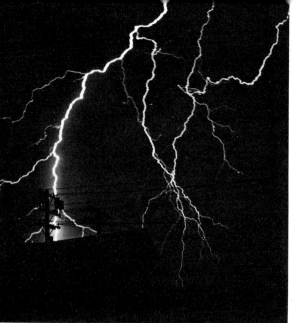

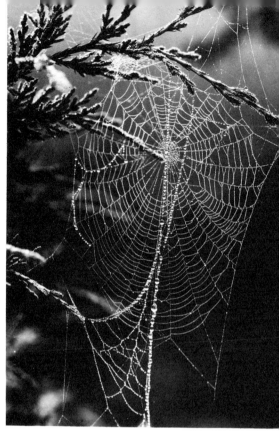

The organisation of nature is patterned rather than linear (see the illustration on page 10). Similar shapes in nature may be seen in lightning flashing, like thought, across the sky, the interconnecting strands of a spider's web . . .

the way in which his or her thoughts were formed. Between them, they came up with a variety of keys—colours, shapes, 'pictures', 'ideas'—anything but ordered grammar. They learned that grammar and syntax are required *after* the ideas are flowing: that 'good English' is a useful cosmetic rather than the innate nature of the idea.

It was then explained to the children that the hooked nature of words and ideas could be used to show them how their brains actually did think and link thoughts. They were shown a number of patterns consisting of extensively hooked words which formed a network of linked idea-word-images. They were then shown images of neuronal branching and immediately noticed the similarity. The *naturalness* of the similarity was stressed. The children were immensely impressed by the similarities which were presented to them. They had organised their ideas like lightning, like nerve cells, like roots and branches of trees, like chemical bonds, like river deltas . . .

The children were once again asked to prepare a talk for the class. The instructions and materials available were identical. In contrast with their initial response, this time every child chose and used the

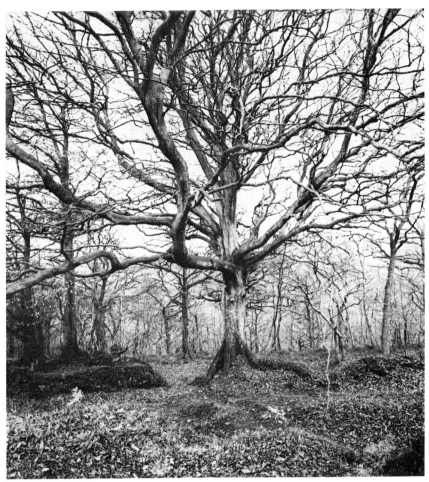

. . . and in the complex branching of a tree (*Frank W. Lane; Frank W. Lane, photograph by Hugh Spencer; Robert Estall*)

largest possible sheet of blank paper and employed a large number of coloured pens. During the half-hour available each child built up a striking mind pattern of the words, ideas, images and linked thoughts in his or her head. They were totally engrossed and disappointed when the time was up. The improvement was remarkable. Their fear of spelling mistakes disappeared (without any increase in them); there was no reluctance. The volume of ideas noted down was on average ten times greater than before. This does not

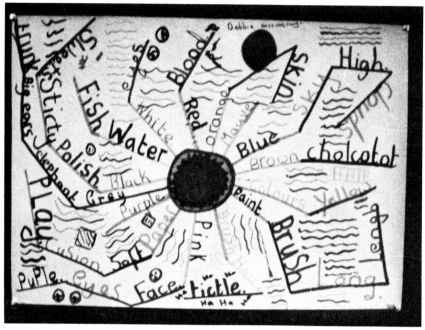

Debbie McCartney's mind pattern picture (*Tony Buzan*)

take into account the amount of colour or number of images used.

When the time came to make their second presentation to the class there was a dramatic increase in confidence, length and interest of the talk. Their mind patterns certainly enabled each child to see more clearly and fully what he or she wanted to say and helped them to present their expanded ideas to the class. Very few children chose the same subject for their second talk although they were free to do entirely what they wished on both occasions. Throughout the second round of talks the level of attention was considerably raised, there was a great deal of laughter, genuine exchange of information took place. Above all there was enthusiasm.

3 Learning about Learning

Education and self-improvement

We are now at a changing point in the history of education. No longer can we think of a classroom as 'thirty kids'. From now on, each teacher should realise that within every child in every class lies an almost unlimited potential.

Traditionally, societies have selected various subjects which were considered important for members of that society and have attempted through various methods to instil this desired knowledge into the minds of the children. The approach has varied, but in general the child has been expected to listen to what was being taught, to note what was being said, to comprehend, to retain, to recall, and finally to re-present in the form of examinations, essays, class response and so on. Throughout this schooling, it has been assumed that the various processes—recognition, understanding, memory, articulation—are somehow 'natural' and that the child simply needed to have the information presented in a reasonable manner to be able to absorb and use it.

Even with the best intentions, however, no society seems to have been able to eliminate the enormous range of problems that everyone experiences with learning. The most common problems noted by people of all societies are as follows:

concentration	boredom
organisation	time pressure
logic	selection
rejection	sequencing
retention	recall
fear	bias
anxiety	environment

studying	note-taking
uncertainty	problem-solving
thinking	creating

The only way to eliminate these problems is to approach education in a new manner. Rather than bombarding the individual with information about various subjects, it is now more important to teach the individual about himself; not to demand that he is a passive receptacle, but to teach him *how* to listen, *how* he understands, *what* is the nature of recall, retention, communication. With this fundamental data the individual is more able to approach any subject with equanimity and enthusiasm rather than fear and foreboding.

It is worth noting that the development of most people is not as 'natural' as has been assumed. New evidence about babies indicates that they have an almost insatiable appetite for learning, and that if they are *allowed* to learn they *will* learn far more than they normally do. What we now accept as normal is in fact a stunted growth for which we are all responsible. Because we assume that what presently *is* is normal, we guide our children to repeat the patterns we have previously experienced. We now need to examine the paths that are open to the child and to allow the child to explore those paths as well as the traditional ones.

Examples abound of people who were effectively squashed at an early stage and who subsequently accepted that they had no ability in certain areas when the truth is that they were probably quite capable. For example, a small girl travelling on the London underground was overheard to say 'Mummy, wouldn't it be marvellous if the train could go so fast that it would be faster than time, because then we could tell Daddy what tomorrow was like!'. The mother's immediate reply was 'Don't be so stupid, of course trains can't go

'If this property of complexity could somehow be transformed into visible brightness . . .' (see p11). 'Le principe du plaisir' by Magritte (*Edward James Foundation, photo: A. C. Cooper,* © *by ADAGP Paris, 1978*)

(overleaf) The pathway traced by dialling a telephone number can be likened to the reflex functions of the brain (*Reproduced by kind permission of 10cc and Hipgnosis; drawing by George Hardie*)

Earthrise: one of a series of photographs that have changed man's perception of himself and his planet (*Picturepoint*)

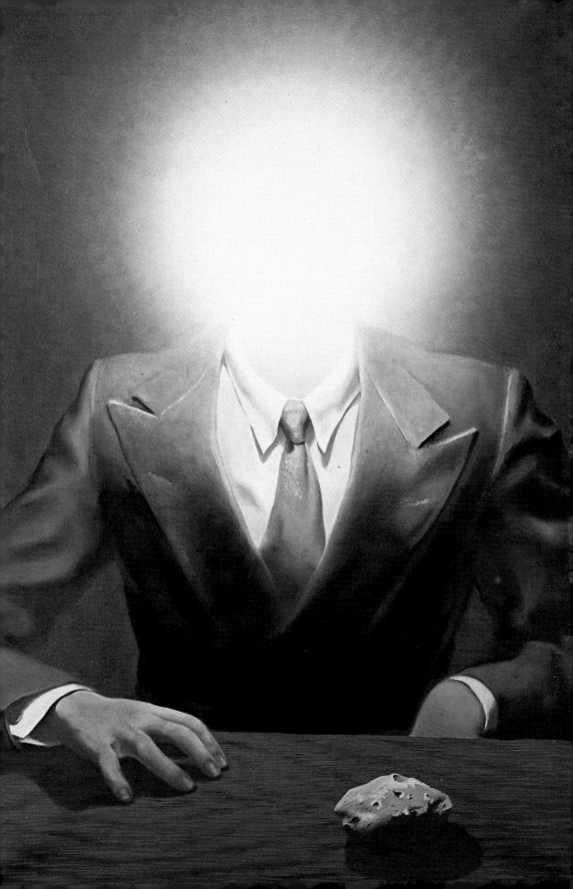

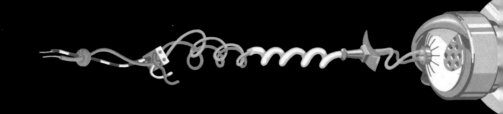
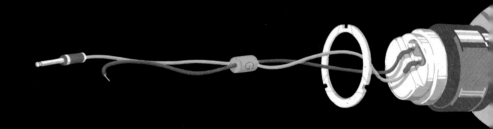

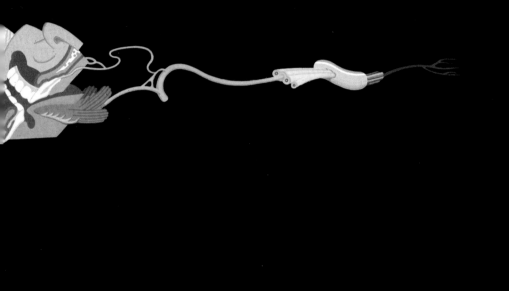
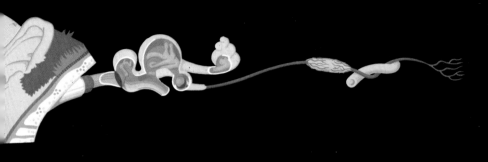
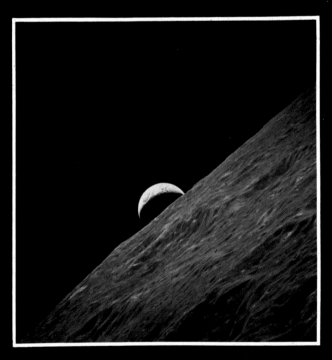

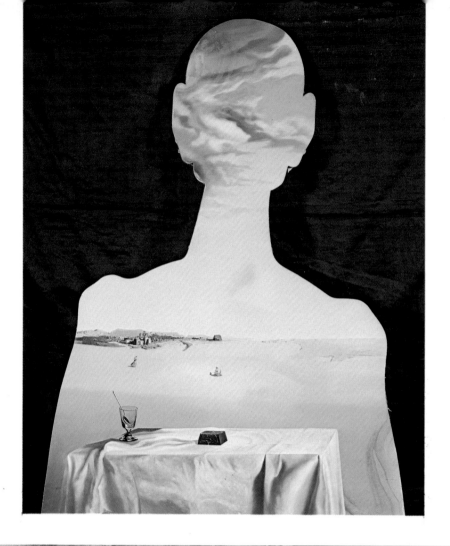

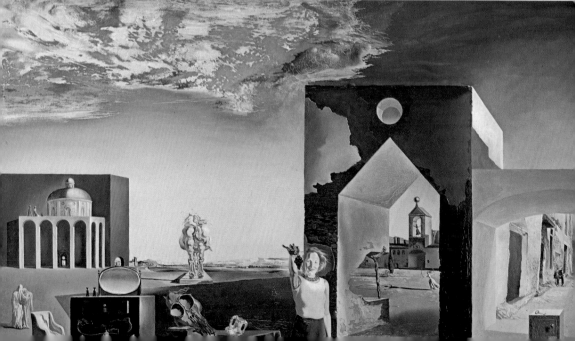

that fast'. The little girl learned, through this 'lesson', that imaginative thinking about time and travel was 'rewarded' with punishment.

In schools and homes the eternal questions why, when, how, where and what are often answered with a short-tempered reply to the effect that the child should not ask stupid questions. (Often the questions are only 'stupid' because the adult cannot answer them.) Such training associates curiosity with punishment and indicates to the child that an inquiring mind is something to avoid.

We hinder the development of a child's mind also when we discourage activities associated with the right hemisphere of the brain (see also Chapter 6). Certain kinds of imaginative thinking, day dreaming, artisan skills, even humour are not held to be as valuable as the more 'academic' or 'intellectual' activities associated with words and numbers. Thus many children who displayed considerable ability in the more unconventional creative areas have often been relegated to the lower streams and an enormous amount of human ability has been undermined.

Even those who have received the encouragement of promotion to university levels often graduate with a singular lack of desire to learn more. The comment is often heard 'I can't understand why he is no longer interested, he has had a good education'. What we have meant by a good education is that the student has been confronted with the information that we thought he should have, not that he has been taught about himself, how to learn and the pleasures that can be derived from learning.

We have also tended to stunt our growth with our traditional assumptions about the measurement and range of human abilities. We have measured 'ability' with IQ and creativity tests that largely assume the score obtained to be absolute. This could not be further from the truth. Many studies now confirm that ability is at least as

'The thing was a spectrum of possibilities from the most remote past to the most remote future – from the most probable to the Most improbable' (see p155). 'Couple with their heads full of clouds – the man' by Salvador Dali (*Edward James Foundation, photo: A. C. Cooper,* © ADAGP Paris, 1978)

The brain contains a vast store of unused and unconscious material that is there for us to draw on. 'Outskirts of paranoia – critical town' by Salvador Dali (*Edward James Foundation, photo: A. C. Cooper,* © ADAGP Paris, 1978)

dependent on environment as heredity and that any score can be drastically altered with appropriate learning.

A study undertaken by the Rehabilitation Research and Training Center in Mental Retardation at the University of Wisconsin has shown that by paying special attention to under-privileged children, IQ scores can be improved by as much as thirty times. Work such as that described in Chapter 2 indicates that measurable changes can be effected in a matter of hours. Any such 'score', therefore, depends not on innate ability, but on the kind of information a subject is given to deal with the mental problems which might confront him.

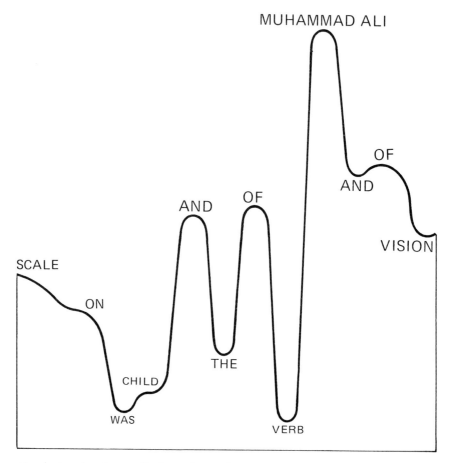

Graph showing the recall of words (see facing page)

The mass of evidence about the human brain, about the potential of the very young and about the inadequacy of our previous teaching and testing methods, leads to a need for a total re-examination of the way in which we approach the nurturing of the human child. We must begin to teach *how* to learn and not *what* to learn alone. We must concentrate on retention and recall, the use of the eyes for reading and taking in information, new approaches to study, an examination of the way in which information itself is structured and in which the information is received, stored and used by the human brain, and the way in which information is transferred from one mind to another. It is also essential that we teach every child all that we currently know about what his mind actually is, and what his mind has the potential to achieve—motivation has long been known to be a prime factor in mental functioning, and the more the child knows about the excellence of himself, the more likely he is to be motivated to a more proper use.

Memory

People can often be overheard explaining just how bad their memories are, and phrases such as 'my memory's not what it used to be', 'I have an awful memory for names and faces', 'I can *never* remember numbers' abound! The truth of the matter is that memory is one of the most amazing aspects of our minds, and that we simply have not understood just how it works or how to use it properly.

First, it is important to understand that memory is not a *single* concept. It is in fact broken down into at least two major parts: recall and retention. Recall is obviously our ability to get out of our brain that which is stored in it, while retention is our ability to actually store the information.

Recall can be divided into two main divisions: recall during learning, and recall after learning. Recall during learning is largely dependent on the time we spend learning. It is known that as time goes on our recall tends to sag in the middle. It is also known that during any learning period we will recall far more of the things that are linked together, and things which are outstanding. Thus if you try to remember the following list of words—scale, on, was, child, and, the, of, verb, Muhammad Ali, and, of, vision—you will find that the beginnings of that list will be recalled, the ends will probably

47

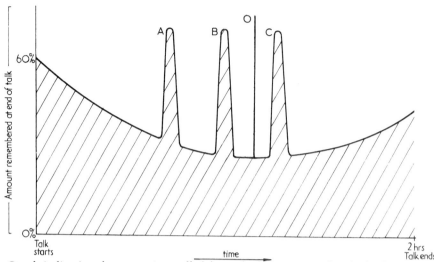

Graph indicating that more is recalled from the beginning and end of a learning period. More is recalled when things are associated or linked (A, B & C) and even more when things are outstanding or unique (O)

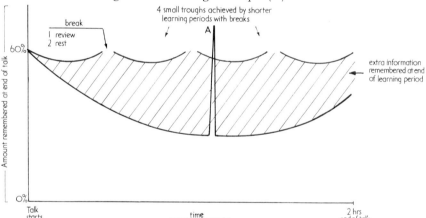

A learning period of 20–40 minutes produces the best relationship between understanding and recalling

be recalled a little bit better, the repeated words—'and', 'of'—will be recalled, as will the outstanding phrase—'Muhammad Ali'. Our recall tends to work like this no matter what the situation, and the longer time goes on the worse the sag in the middle will be.

Once this aspect of our memory is understood, we can change the way in which we organise time during learning, in order to enable the recall to function as well as possible. It is important to note here that

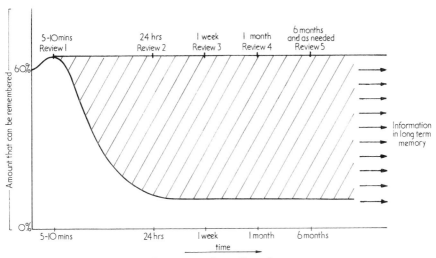

Graph showing the effect of review and recall on long-term memory

recall and understanding are *not* the same concept. It is possible to understand completely what one is reading or learning and to be forgetting, all the time, what one is understanding! It is therefore essential that recall and understanding be organised so as to work in the most harmonious way.

It transpires that the best time period for recall and understanding to work together is approximately 20–40 minutes. Thus if a person wishes recall to be high while understanding remains high, it is essential that he organises his time in this way. Once recall *during* learning has improved, it is essential to make sure that recall *after* learning is improved.

It is normally assumed that when we have finished learning, our forgetting process immediately sets in and that within a week or so most of the information has disappeared. The surprising truth of the matter is that immediately after learning, whether or not we consciously review, our recall rises for a few minutes! The reason for this can be seen when we realise that once the brain has taken a body of information in, it needs a little while in order to let that information 'sink in'. This 'sinking in' process really means that the mind is organising, associating, linking, and putting into a more final form all the information that it has acquired during the learning period.

49

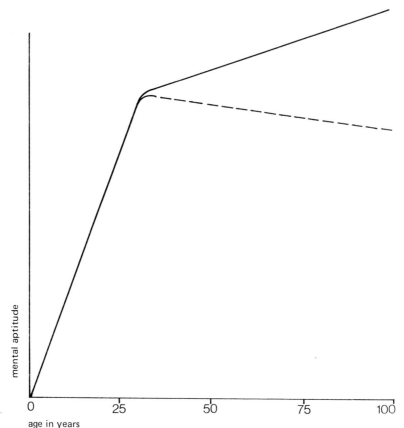

age in years

Graph showing the general loss of mental ability with age after 25 (dotted line) and the rise of ability amongst mentally stimulated aged people (unbroken line)

Having realised that there is an enormous drop shortly after the little rise, the next important task is to prevent the drop from recurring. This is accomplished by using a proper review method. Once again it is essential to understand the nature of the mind, its recall and its reviewing techniques before deciding to review material learnt. As with recall during learning, it is necessary to review at the best and most appropriate time. This turns out to be a fairly simple formula: if for example you have studied for one hour, in order to keep that recall high it is necessary to review approximately ten minutes after the hour, approximately one day after that, and then at periods of a week, two weeks, a month, and six months. These review periods need not be more than perhaps two or three minutes.

If they are done properly recall will be maintained at the highest level, and new learning will be made far more easy.

If we nurture recall during learning, and look after recall after learning, our total recall of the information we have learnt will be almost 100% of what we desire. This compares with the normal 1–10%—a staggering difference.

This information about recall can be related to the problem of decline of mental abilities with human ageing. It has been assumed that as a person gets older his mind gets worse. Psychologists' graphs abound proving that after the age of 18–25 it is more or less all over as far as our minds' mental abilities are concerned. The peak is reached at 25, after which a steady decline is seen. These studies are supported by a number of arguments. Firstly, the argument that the brain loses brain cells after the age of 20; secondly, that whenever studies have been done following people through their lives they have shown a gradual decline in mental ability; and thirdly, that when studies have been done which pick people at 0, at 10, 20, 30, 40, 50, 60, 70 years of age, again declines are shown by the older members of the group.

Fortunately each one of these arguments can be contradicted. The argument that the brain loses cells as it gets older can be counteracted by the arguments put forward by Professor Rosenzweig which show that it is not the number of brain cells that is important, but the number of inter-connections between them. Rosenzweig successfully showed that stimulation, at no matter what age it occurred, increased the number of connections between the brain cells at a far greater rate than the actual loss of brain cells. Rosenzweig has thus shown that it is possible for the brain to become more intelligent as it grows older (see Chapter 1).

The arguments concerning decline with age can both be put aside when one realises that the people being tested *were* declining with age because of their environment, not by a 'natural' process.

What normally happens to a person between the ages of 20 and 25? He 'finishes his education' (an extraordinary phrase in itself) and *settles down* (not *up*!). If a mind is placed in this situation, where it is no longer required to learn new information at the previous rate, and where its basic life becomes a matter of routine, it will obviously gradually lose some of its abilities to perform mentally. This loss will then be reflected on any graph testing mental agility. If however, the mind is not prevented from learning, and is continually encouraged to expand and use its mental facilities, it will continue to improve into old age.

If a person does not review, allowing his information to slide away from him as soon as it comes in, obviously the mind has very little to deal with, and has little to help it deal with new information. If, however, it allows itself to review and maintain its information, it has more to deal with and more to connect to new information that comes in. The situation reflects the biblical phrase 'to him that hath shall be given, and to him that hath not even that little which he hath shall be taken away'.

In addition to this new information on recall, much has come to light concerning the other aspect of our memory: retention. There is now enough evidence available to suggest that our retention may be far more near to perfect than we had previously assumed. Among the areas of evidence are the following:

Dreams. Everyone has experienced at some time or another a dream in which a person or an event from their distant past recurs in perfect clarity during the course of the dream. This suggests that there is a vast store of unused and unconscious material that is there for us to draw on if necessary.

Death-type experiences. A number of people who have fallen off cliffs or been in head-on collisions report that for the split second before they became unconscious, and while assuming that their life had come to an end, their entire life ran before them like a film. They report that the split second seemed like an age, that time seemed to slow down completely and that their entire life in every detail, raced before their eyes.

Perfect memories. Perhaps the most famous of these is that of the Russian 'S' (see Chapter 4). 'S' had such a perfect memory that if he were asked if he could remember 25 June twenty years ago, he would reply something to the tune of 'What time on 25 June?' 'S' was able to remember not only his normal day-to-day experiences but also complicated formulas that he had memorised but did not understand. As many as twenty years later he was able to reproduce these formulas perfectly. There are a number of other people like 'S', and all indications are that their minds are no different from any other minds; it is just that their initial training seemed to set them off on a self-programme of recording and recalling everything that happened to them.

Language. We all use language as something which comes as second nature to us. The minute we stop to think about it however it sheds light on our enormous memory capacity. Every word, phrase and sentence that we either speak or listen to is being 'recalled' by our minds. Few people find themselves continually interrupting those speaking to them with 'Hold on a minute, I can't remember that word'. In other words, as everyone else's communication pours into us, our minds record and recall it instantly, as well as putting it into a meaningful context. This again indicates that even in normal functioning, the mind is doing the most extraordinary memory feats.

Random memories. Experiences are often reported where a person either sees, hears, or smells, something which stimulates a memory from years ago. One of the most common of these experiences is the return to a person's first school. Entering an old room; smelling the old canteen smells; all of these things can trigger off, perfectly, recall of events that occurred sometimes as many as seventy years ago. These random occurrences again suggest that there may be many other stored memories which simply are awaiting the trigger to bring them back to life again.

Memory techniques. There are special memory techniques, mnemonics, which enable people to remember as many as a thousand items in random order backwards and forwards. Once a person has been trained in these mnemonic techniques, his ability to remember such lists is virtually infallible. Once again this ability to produce perfect recall suggests that the ability to store may be perfect.

Physiological structure of the brain. Work done by Rosenzweig and Professor Anokhin in Russia indicates that the number of interconnections available to the human brain is a number 1 followed by about ten million kilometres of noughts! If our brain is able to make this number of physical interconnections, there is a strong possibility that it can also make the same number of mental connections. Professor Rosenzweig has estimated that the brain could take in ten

E.B.—D

new bits of information *every* second, for an entire life-time and still not be half full!

Vision

In addition to this encouraging information about memory, there is additional and similar information about our eyes and their ability to absorb information. The rapid rise of the speed reading schools was evidence of man's desire to use his eyes more efficiently. These schools were correct in their assumption that man could in fact take in information more rapidly and more efficiently at the same time, but were incorrect in the way that they attempted to bring about this increased capacity.

The average speed reading school guaranteed to increase a person's ability by perhaps 50% and gave a number of speeding up exercises over a period of as many as ten weeks, graphing progress. The error that these schools made, and the reason for their gradual decline, was that the person's average range of abilities goes from his normal speed, which is in fact usually his lowest, to a speed which is somewhere between 50% and 100% above that that he normally uses. What the speed reading schools were therefore doing was increasing a person's ability to the maximum of his normal range, instead of having his normal range permanently extended. When the speed reading course had been completed and the person's motivation had obviously declined a little, the speed declined with the loss of motivation and the person generally reverted to his previous habits.

The latest information on our eyes suggests that they are able to take in the information on which they focus and are *also* able to see information in a fairly wide area around that on which they are pin-pointedly focusing. Making use of this increased visual awareness, a person can direct his mind to select those pieces of information in an entire page which are relevant to the questions he is asking of the material, and can therefore read at speeds comfortably approaching two to five thousand words a minute with virtually 100% of the comprehension desired.

In certain cases, a metronome can be used to pace the eyes at even higher speeds, especially for purposes of review. Once a mind has gone through a given book, most of the information will probably be retained somewhere in the deeper recesses of the brain. Training at high-speed, visual selective scanning, by the use of the rhythmic beat of the metronome, can enable a person to review a book already read at speeds of up to 30,000 words per minute.

It becomes apparent that if we realise the different ways in which our eyes can function we can apply them for different purposes. The intake of information therefore is no longer restricted to a word by word, line by line, plodding along, but can be adjusted to the particular purpose at hand. If the individual wishes to read at 100 words per minute he can adjust his eyes to do so. If however he wishes to read between 500 and 1,000 words per minute he can use his knowledge about his perceptual processes to attain those speeds. And finally, if he wishes to use more advanced selection and scanning techniques, and if these techniques are appropriate, then he can acquire speeds in the tens of thousands with adequate comprehension for the task at hand. Thus the definition of reading changes to be more comprehensive than it has previously been, and the range of abilities of the reader is correspondingly increased.

Expanding this point into our general perception, it is now known that our eyes can see much farther than has previously been assumed, and can be used more miscroscopically than has been assumed. Our error in the past has been to assume that what was normal was the definition of the capacity. What is now apparent is that what is normal is most certainly what is, but that the boundaries of 'what is' can be extended. This applies to our everyday seeing, as well as to our more academic reading and studying. If eyes are used more accurately, if they are exercised, if the individual tries to see more in everything that he does see, their ability will be increased correspondingly.

The advantage of this is that the clearer the images entering the brain, the 'clearer' the memory of those images will be, and the more proficient the general functioning of the mind will be. It can be seen then that perception aids memory, that memory aids learning, that learning aids perception. We therefore have a cycle in which, if each element is improved, the others automatically improve.

Extending the information about our eyes into the more general field of technical study, it is found that, by adding information about the way our mind 'sets' itself, we can also help to increase effectiveness while taking in information. Mental set, the 'direction' we give to our mind, is becoming an increasingly important factor in research concerning the mind. It is also particularly important nowadays in sport, where many of the leading athletes give themselves a mental set before competing.

It is found almost invariably that those athletes who do give themselves a realistic mental set do better than those who do not. The situation is similar in study. If the person sets himself a reasonable amount to study, sets a reasonable time in which to study that amount, and sets the aims and goals for that particular reading, far more will be gained from the reading than would have been gained otherwise. What is happening here is that the mind is organising itself beforehand for the task it is about to accomplish. The better the mind is organised, the better the results of the given task will be. By better we do not simply mean 5–10%, but often 100% improvement.

Mind patterns

Our inherent abilities are greater than we have thought, our memory can most definitely be improved far beyond current levels, and the ability of our eyes to take in information is greater than we thought.

A mind pattern on the subject of memory

In addition to this, and as indicated in the previous chapter, the way in which we handle our language can also be improved. It has been traditionally assumed that man was a language and linear thinker. For this reason most of our writing and recording has been in sentence form using lines and lists. It is now apparent that our minds do not generally or normally think in this way, but that they think in images, key words and linked patterns. These patterns also tend to make use of most of our different senses.

These 'mind patterns' are in effect tracings by the hand of images and linked pieces of information occurring naturally in the mind. The relevance of these patterns can be seen when looking at the enormous improvement in performance of the children who substituted mind patterns for their traditional method of approaching and organising the information in their minds. The patterns, based on our knowledge that each piece of information has many hooks, have enormous application.

Most of our problems in organising, sequencing, logic, and ordering of information stem from the fact that we try to force it into line and list sequences when really its 'order' is far more organic. We have tended to confuse the word logic with the concept of list order. What we really mean when we use logic in the colloquial sense is 'associated

A mind pattern may help in recalling a person's name

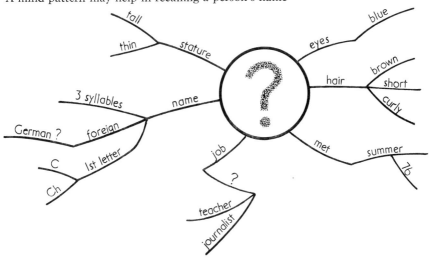

in a reasonable way'. And this, of course, is what the pattern enables us to do. From the basis of such pattern the information can be represented in a linked and understandable manner. Thus the application of the patterns becomes appropriate whenever a person wishes to re-order any information.

Patterns can be used, for instance, in the preparation of speeches. All the thoughts that come into a person's head about the subject he wishes to speak can be jotted down in a pattern form. When they are all organised, each branch can be given an order depending on whether the speaker wishes to use that branch first, second or third and so on. In presenting the speech the information will therefore flow in an ordered, linked and organised form, which can be varied if the circumstance demands it. Such a speech will also tend to be more natural and flowing, because the rigidity that often accompanies a list-like speech will be gone, and a spontaneity will be substituted. The amount of time spent preparing such a speech will also be considerably less than the previous method, because patterned thoughts tend to flow more rapidly and efficiently than falsely ordered list-thoughts.

Patterns can also be used for the generation of creative ideas. What usually happens when we try to generate a large number of creative ideas is that we start with a burst and gradually trail off. This is because each thought tends to require that we go to another area for the next thought. With a pattern, each thought *encourages* other thoughts, and each of those others encourages even more, so that we start off with a burst and end with an even greater burst.

Note-taking is another area where patterns are useful. Notes taken in the normal linear form tend to be 'all the same'. This means that when we come to review them nothing stands out as unique or memorable and the important information is lost in the maze of general words. The pattern technique of taking notes enables the important information to be emphasized either by position, colour shape or form. Each pattern note could also be unique to itself, and therefore will be more memorable as an individual entity. Experiments done in this area have shown that people taking pattern notes take, on average, one-fifth of the normal volume of notes, one-tenth of the time to review those notes, and score between 80% and 100% on tests testing their recall of what was noted, as opposed to the normal 50% to 70% on the more linear notes.

Rather than forcing children into the more complicated and unnatural grammatical structures into which we normally force them, they can be encouraged, as the children at Poplar school were, to spray out their ideas, images and colours, in a natural generation of ideas. Once they have done this they will feel less fear when confronted with language, and will tend to learn, note, remember and create with far more ease, readiness and enjoyment than they would otherwise do. In fact a semi-literate child can become literate in just a few weeks if he is given encouragement of this sort.

Pattern application can in fact be applied to virtually any situation where the person wishes to use his mind applied to language. Therefore patterns can be used in problem solving, analysis, planning, report writing, book writing, brain storming and meetings. It can also be seen that the patterning technique makes use of both the left and the right hemispheres of our brain. Ornstein pointed out that the left side of our brain tends to organise language, number, analysis and criticism, whereas the right side of our brain organises and takes responsibility for rhythm, spatial awareness, colour, shape and form (see Chapter 6). Normal notes, of course, make use of only one side of the brain. The pattern note makes use of both sides. Language is used, but is used in the context of colours, shapes, images and forms. As Ornstein predicted, if each side of the brain is used, both sides will produce more than if only one side is used. Therefore the increase is greater than simply the sum of the two halves. This has been found with patterns, as once again can be seen from the Poplar experiment. Once the children were allowed to use both sides of their brain, in conjunction with specific information about the way language does naturally work for them, they produced much more than twice the volume in a given period. In many cases the increases in actual number of significant key words and images were as much as fifty times.

In this chapter a few pieces of basic information have been given about what we now know concerning the potential of our minds. If this basic information is applied, children can be—and have already been—taken from the bottom of the class to the top. Perhaps more important than this simple accomplishment criterion is the fact that anyone introduced to the magnificent potential of his/her mind tends to become more enthusiastic about words like 'reading', 'study', 'learning' and 'education'. In the past these words have become associated with regimentation, boredom, fear and stress. From now on they can be associated with enthusiasm, accomplishment, encouragement and enjoyment.

If this information is made generally available, then the dreams of many of the fore-thinking educators will be realised. Education will become what they have always wished, a situation in which individuals approach information with zest, and in which teachers will be guides through various mazes rather than perpetrators of intellectual punishment for non-accomplishment. Such an approach will also render as prehistoric those techniques which assume to test abilities in order to determine future results. In the future, tests will be used only to indicate where the system has so far failed, to show a person how to use that part of the brain which on the test is revealed as not yet awakened, rather than already dead.

It is significant that at the moment absenteeism and truancy are on the increase in the schools of many Western countries. In many large cities such as London, the percentage of children staying away each day from school is as high as 30%. When children are encouraged to use their minds, rather than being punished for being ignorant about them, this discouraging trend will be reversed.

4 Beyond Pavlov

Two great Russian researchers

The original giant of Russian psychology was Ivan Pavlov, who in 1904 received the first Nobel Prize in psychology. Pavlov is renowned for his development of the conditional reflex theory based on stimulus to the brain and a corresponding response from the body.

In his initial experiments, Pavlov used dogs as his subjects. He began by ringing a bell, and immediately after having rung the bell he gave the dogs food which they liked. He repeated this process, measuring the amount of saliva that the dogs formed in their mouths each time the bell rang. The further the experiment progressed, the more saliva the dogs produced at the ringing of the bell. In the final stages of the experiment, Pavlov was able to ring the bell, produce no food at all, and still observe that the dogs produced an amount of

Ivan Pavlov with the personnel of the Physiology Chair of the Military and Medical Academy, Petrograd, 1914 (*Barnaby's Picture Library*)

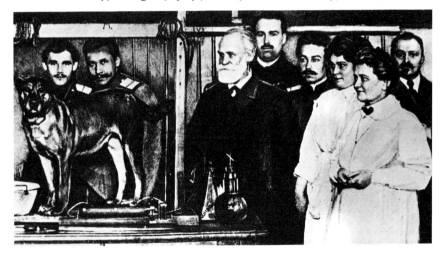

saliva equivalent to that they would have produced if they had been given food.

What Pavlov established with this experiment was the fact that the brain programmes the rest of the body to respond, based on its experience. This also established that the brain had a certain freedom of choice to select the stimulation in the environment to which it wished to react, and then to send instructions to the body to react in a certain way.

In recent years Pavlov's major student, Professor Pyotr Anokhin, has taken Pavlov's work much farther. Anokhin has shown that not only does the brain have freedom of choice, but that each single neuron in the brain has also a great freedom of choice as to which connections it will make. Anokhin has also established that this choice is based on feeding back to the neuron the actual results of the action it has suggested should take place.

In order to establish this fact, Anokhin devised the following experiment: he placed tiny recording electrodes in the individual neurons of the conscious human brain. He then gave the person a choice of different kinds of cups. In one situation a cup was empty, and in the other situation the cup was full of tea. The subject of the

Professor Anokhin

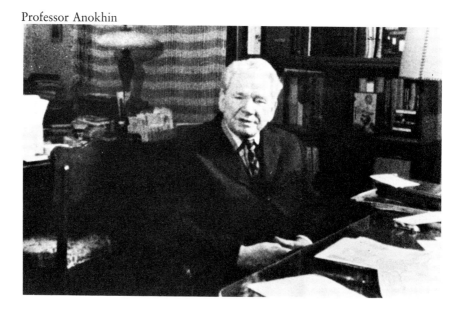

experiment was asked to raise the cup to her lips as if drinking tea. What Anokhin observed was that when the cup was empty the neurons gave off one kind of electrical signal, indicating that a certain set of connections had been made. But when the cup was full of tea, the signal was different. This time the brain had had different expectations and had already experienced different results. And so when the cup was full of tea the same neurons made different connections as indicated by a different electrical signal.

From this Professor Anokhin concluded that each single neuron, each one ten billionth part of the human brain, has tremendous choice. He also established that the neuron makes this choice not by a simple stimulus, but based on the stimulus, experience, *and* expectation.

Carrying his experiments further, Professor Anokhin noted that if the expectation of the neuron is raised, each neuron involved in the mental pathway for the activity changes its connections. In fact the more that was expected from the neurons the more they responded. Contrary to the normal assumptions that the brain does not 'grow', Professor Anokhin's work showed that if the brain were expected to become involved in more complicated activity, the individual neurons of the brain grew more connections. The conclusions that he reached,

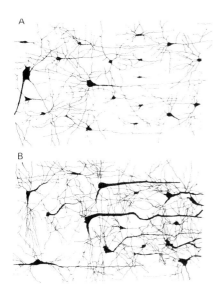

Tracings from the same region of a human baby's brain showing increased connections: A at three months, B at twenty-four months

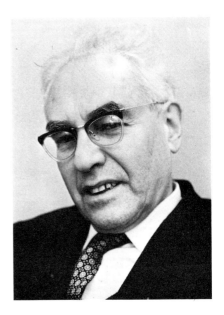

Professor Luria (*Novosti Press Agency*)

therefore, were that the more one expected from the brain in general, the more the individual neurons would grow extensions, and therefore the more 'heavy' or 'dense' the brain would become.

These conclusions are confirmed by the work of Professor Rosenzweig (see Chapter 1) who also found that when increasing the stimulus in the environment of rats, he observed a corresponding increase in the number of interconnections within the rats' brains. Professor Rosenzweig's rats, no matter what their age, showed a significant increase in the density of their brains after they had been introduced to situations in which they were required to be more active, creative, and intelligent.

These findings are further confirmed by the work of Tony Buzan at Poplar. When the expectation of the children who were performing mental feats was raised, the amount that they produced was correspondingly greater.

Professor Anokhin went even further, developing a new theory called the 'Function System Theory', which suggested that the brain did not work in individual bits, nor as a general whole, but as a series of interlinked and interlaced systems.

As Anokhin was the great student of Pavlov, so was Professor

Luria the great student of Professor Anokhin. The late Professor Luria was one of the most famous psychologists in the world, and following is an interview in which he explained, in his own 'English', the basic elements of the functional system as originally devised by Professor Anokhin. In the interview Professor Luria discussed some of the implications and ramifications of the theory:

'During the last forty years my collaborators and I took part in a creation of the new branch of science, neuropsychology. What is really neuropsychology? It is a new branch of science located between psychology and neurology. You can say that neuropsychology is the application of scientifically psychological methods to the diagnosis of brain lesions, and for rehabilitation.

'But *why* neuropsychology? You see, the last decades were the decades of a tremendous progress in neurology and neurosurgery. When I began to work with the famous neurosurgeon Professor Bourdenko, the mortality from brain tumour operations was about 60-70%. Now the mortality is only 6-7%. The people survive. But to make a precise operation you have to make a topical diagnosis of the site of the lesion as early as possible and here are some troubles, because neurologists have really a very limited range of possibilities for analysing the patient, for analysing his sensitivity.

'The very complicated parts of the human brain that are special to human beings and which deal with our behaviour processes don't "say" anything for a neurologist. They are called the "mute" zones. But I'm really sure that no mute zones of the brain exist. Neurologists and scientists are simply hard of hearing! We have to understand the voices of these complicated parts of the brain and to understand that we have to create special tests. And that is why neuropsychology came to life.

'But how do we work? What are the principles of neuropsychology? First, the history. There are two lines of study: about one hundred years ago the French surgeon Broker had showed that the lesions of the lower part of the pre-motor zone results in a defect of speech although the patient can understand speech. Thirteen years later a German psychiatrist, Vernike, showed that the lesion of the posterior parts of the left temporal zone brings a reverse phenomenon, the patient can't understand speech, but he can speak! So it was supposed that there was a centre for speech, a centre for speech understanding and so on. In the seventies of the nineteenth century there were a lot of attempts to find hundreds of centres; centres for writing, centres for calculation, centres for memory and so on. It was the concept of strict localisation of function. But it was found after about fifty years that such centres don't exist, and another idea came into being: the idea that the brain is working as a whole.

'But this was a mistake too, because the brain cortex is a differentiated apparatus, and every part of the brain seems to take its own part in the organisation of mental processes.

'So a crisis was seen and we had to overcome this crisis, the struggle between strict localisation and the holistic approach. Now how did we overcome this crisis? We had to revise the concept of function and to revise the concept of localisation. What *is* this "local" function? It turns out that we have a double understanding of "function". First the function is supposed to be a function of tissue. For instance the retina of the eye has a function to react to light, and the apparatus of our ear has a function to react to sound. Both are functions of special tissues. But this understanding is not adequate enough for our complete understanding of "function". Function should be understood as a function *system*—as a result of the whole system of events.

'Let us take breathing. Of course breathing is a function, but it's a very complex, very complicated function. It is really a function system. The goal of breathing is to bring our oxygen to the alveoli of our lungs, but breathing is not *located* in the alveoli. To breath you have to use the muscles of your diaphragm but if we anaesthetize these muscles your intercostal muscles take over, and if we also anaesthetize these then your throat and mouth muscles take over. So the system does not depend on one set of tissue, it is not invariant, but is a function *system*.

'This idea was originated by our outstanding physiologist, the successor to Pavlov, Professor Anokhin. And now we think that most psychological functions are not functions in the first sense of the word, not functions of tissue, but are function systems. Perception, calculation, writing, speaking, they're function systems which are composed by interrelations of different parts of the brain. That is our revision of the concept of function.

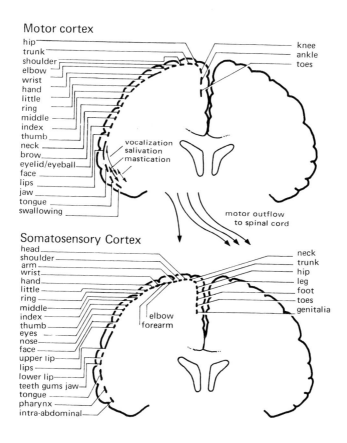

Motor cortex

hip
trunk
shoulder
elbow
wrist
hand
little
ring
middle
index
thumb
neck
brow
eyelid/eyeball
face
lips
jaw
tongue
swallowing

knee
ankle
toes

vocalization
salivation
mastication

motor outflow
to spinal cord

Somatosensory Cortex

head
shoulder
arm
wrist
hand
little
ring
middle
index
thumb
eyes
nose
face
upper lip
lips
lower lip
teeth gums jaw
tongue
pharynx
intra-abdominal

elbow
forearm

neck
trunk
hip
leg
foot
toes
genitalia

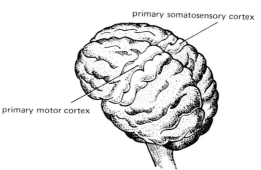

primary somatosensory cortex

primary motor cortex

A plan of the brain illustrating the concept of strict localisation, with the motor cortex 'instructing' the muscles of the opposite side of the body and the somatosensory cortex dealing with impulses from the skin. These days a more wholeistic view of the brain is accepted

'Our second revision is of the concept of localisation. Functions can and must be strictly localised, but function systems are distributed in the brain and *not* localised. So we have to try to find out how are they distributed in the brain cortex, and what role is played by every part of the brain in the fulfilment or realisation of such functions. The best example I can do is to use the process of writing. I could also use as well speech, computation, problem solving or perception.

'What is necessary to write down a word? Firstly, you have to analyse the sounds which you have afterwards to write. They are called phonemes, these units of sound. For instance "b" and "p" play a role in differentiation of the sense of the words "bull" and "pull". So you have to single out phonemes, and only then can you write, but this function has to do with the posterior parts of the left temporal zone which is an acoustic analyzer. And if you have a breakdown of this zone, the man can't write. But to differentiate phonemes is not enough. To write you have to help this differentiation to make clear sounds by the use of your tongue. If you give me a complicated word, for instance "catastrophe", you have to repeat "ca-ta-strophe", using your tongue, and then the contents of the sounds becomes clear. They made an experiment with school children, the class was divided into half, and one half wrote with repetition of the words, and the other half with their mouths closed. The second half made six times more mistakes than the first, showing that the part of the brain was necessary which was involved in actually making the sounds.

'So if I see a certain kind of mistake, for instance for "dum" he writes "lum", that is a symptom of one special part of the brain is disturbed, and for another kind of mistake, then another special part.

'The third component in writing is to transfer the phonemes into letters, and that is to arrange spaciously the letters. Let us take three letters, b, d and p. They all have a semi-circle and a line, but your intention is to write here and here to left and here in the other direction. Now if the third part of the cortex, the parietal-occipital part, is destroyed, then the patient is unable to make this spatial analysis, and he won't understand what is to go to the right and to the left, and that is why for this patient b and d are indistinguishable, the mistakes he makes in writing are very different from mistakes which may refer to other kinds of patients, but that's still not the end.

'To write, you don't write only letters, you write words. It is a sequence of phonemes and letters. You have to shift from one letter to the second to the third and you have to build your writing as a kinetic melody. This process is provided by quite a different zone, the pre-motor zone, and if the pre-motor zone is disturbed the patient can understand and differentiate phonemes and letters, but the sequence of the writing, the fluency, is disturbed.

'And last but not least, you don't write letters or words, you write composition. Letters to your friends and so on. That means that you have a plan of your writing, a programme, and you have to pay attention to the development of this programme. Now for this goal-making and programme-making process, the frontal lobes are responsible.

'I remember a patient who wrote a letter "Dear Professor, I want to tell you, that I want to tell you, that I want to tell you . . ." and nothing else for four pages! That is the symptom of the front lobe region. Now you can understand that writing can be disturbed with every disturbance of the whole left hemisphere of the brain. But the part, the rule of every part of this hemisphere is different, and so we can use the style of the defects of the writing as symptoms which have a topical significance. So if my assistant comes to me and tells me a patient has lost his writing, I say to him it's not enough, tell me what *kind* of factors are disturbed. *How* is his writing disturbed?

'So the goal of neuropsychology is to single out factors underlying the complicated psychological processes. In the last 40 years we have studies similarly in reading, speaking, understanding of speech, problem solving, and now we can use the whole battery of psychological experiments for local diagnosis of brain lesions.

'What other significance has this system for the problems of recovery and rehabilitation? Well, if you start with an approach of strict localisation, and you already know that when cerebral cells are destroyed they don't regenerate, the outlook is pretty pessimistic— the loss of function is a loss forever. But if a function is a function *system*, things are much more optimistic. You can reconstruct the function system and use different parts of the brain which are preserved.

'For example, if a patient has lost his ability to differentiate sounds, we can use other processes. We include visual analysis and the other senses. We use the potentialities of the brain which are different from the one damaged, and we use the mechanisms of these to replace a damaged system. It's a very hard task, it's humane work, and terribly, terribly significant work. That's why half of our work we use for diagnostics and the second half of our work we use for the rehabilitation of the results of the defects.

'Apart from all this is the tremendous significance of neuropsychology for our theoretical psychological concepts. I am quite sure that in 50 years psychological science will be very different from what we have now. We don't yet understand the brain's psychological processes, but with the help of neuropsychology we shall construct a *whole* psychology which will sensibly include every kind of human activity.

'Actually all these ideas started with Professor Vygotsky who died 40 years ago when he was 37. But his influence remains perhaps half a century. The whole concept of function systems and of factor analysis of the components underlying every psychological process was initially his, and as I said, will change the whole face of the scientific psychology in the next decade.

'One last point—I think I would like to make the statement that all our intellectual processes are processes which are *inside*, but if the brain is damaged you have to give the patient *external* help, exteriorize step by step. We have to record it, and the next period make it interiorized again. If you want only one example, I asked a patient to tell me the history of his brain wound which he got in the war time. Many ideas came to the patient, but very irregularly. "I was wounded", "I am working on rehabilitation", "I was operated", "I was in the hospital", but he can't make it, the plan, come together. Then I give him a different instruction: "You have a series of different cards. Please write your ideas on every card, independently of the sequence, then you have a series of cards on the table and you can arrange these cards in a sequence and you have a story."

'So applying the external help using, instead of inner processes, external processes, you can count the recovery of the programmed action afterwards. But it's very slow. The patient can eventually use less and less help and more and more put it in his head. And to a certain limit he can interiorize. It *is* a way to recover, and that's why using adequate methods of rehabilitation we are very optimistic for the possibility of gaining the recovery of mental trace.

'You know our Nicholas Ostrovsky, the famous writer. He was very ill, but with his will he managed the possibility to write compositions. We have dozens of such Ostrovskys, but even more terrible cases, where not the extremities, not the hands or the feet or the legs are disturbed, but the *brain* is disturbed. But now we know we can help the brain-damaged patient to use the potentialities, the inner potentialities of the brain to apply outer, external schemes and reconstruct the lost activities.

'And finally, what about the brain organisation of the will? I can answer you. If the frontal lobes are preserved, then the patient can work and make hard work to rescue these functional systems. But if the frontal lobes are damaged, then he has lost his power to plan, to make programmes, to pay attention, to have the feed forward and feed back. In other words he has lost his will.

'The human brain is a socially organized capacity to create motives, plans, programme and control, and this has to do with the frontal lobes of man. This is the most important part of this wonderful, unique, unique mechanism we call the human brain.'

The work by Professor Luria is already having wide ranging and extremely beneficial social results. Apart from the obvious applications to brain damaged or retarded people, Professor Luria's findings can be applied to the normal teaching of basic processes. His work with the different mental systems of human beings, has shown that where certain difficulties exist, they need not be considered as absolute.

For example, if a child in school is experiencing particular difficulty with either reading, writing, mathematics, speaking, communicating, or remembering, he need no longer be considered as definitely unintelligent, or incapable in the given area of his disability. What is required is a thorough investigation of the reasons for the difficulties that the child is experiencing. If the reasons are not to be found in the family or emotional background of the child, they may well be found to be minor malfunctions in part of the brain's general system. If these malfunctions can be defined, other ways of teaching the child to deal with the particular mental concept can readily be made available. In this way all children will be enabled to develop more completely, and the unfortunate categorising by hierarchical ability will no longer be the yardstick by which children are measured.

In addition to his work with brain damaged people, Professor Luria is also renowned for the work that he has done with people possessing special abilities. The most famous of these is the Russian 'S'. 'S' was a Russian journalist who was discovered in the 1920s. His editor had noticed that at all the briefing sessions, 'S' had failed to take any notes. When 'S' was questioned and criticised for this he became embarrassed, and seemed to have no understanding of why anyone *would* take notes. It was found on further questioning that he was able to remember *everything* that he had been told. He was quickly introduced to Professor Luria who immediately ran a series of tests on his memory. The results were astounding.

On all the standard memory tests, the capacity and durability of his memory was virtually perfect! Professor Luria after years of investigation, uncovered the facts that 'S' had always had a phenomenal memory, and that he could even remember his emotional reactions while in his pram. In addition to a phenomenal memory, his senses also tended to blend things. So that whenever he heard words he would not only have a mental picture of the word, but would associate with each word a different sound, a different smell, 'feel', 'movement' and so on.

'S' was also able to solve conceptional problems by 'imagining' them. He also reported that he was often able to eliminate pain by forming a perfect image of the pain in his mind, and then imagining that the image was gradually disappearing to the horizon. When the image finally disappeared over the horizon, the pain disappeared with it! 'S' was further able to change his temperature, once again by making mental images in his mind of the kind of temperature he wanted to be in. If he felt like being hot, that is he felt like raising his temperature, he simply imagined that he was in a very hot place. If he wanted to lower his temperature, he imagined that he was on the Arctic Circle.

What is significant about the memory of 'S' is firstly that it was so comprehensive, secondly that it was based on perfect imagination, and thirdly that because of it 'S' was able to perform other mental feats. Unfortunately at the time not enough was known about how to select and reject from memory, so his amazing memory became a problem for him in that he could not forget even if he wanted to.

What is ultimately significant about the mind of 'S' is that it was an average mind. It was simply that at an early age, his mind 'triggered' onto the way in which memory functioned, and he simply functioned in that way for the remainder of his life. His story, exhaustively written up by Professor Luria in his book *The Mind of a Mnemonist*, comprehensively covers his life, as well as explaining the various techniques and approaches he used for solving memory problems, solving conceptual problems, changing his temperature, and projecting his images. Professor Luria's book is virtually a 'how to do it manual' on acquiring a phenomenal memory.

The positive work of Professor Anokhin and Professor Luria is made even more positive by a major finding from Professor Anokhin's last two years of research. Observing that the more we expect the more the neurons will respond, Professor Anokhin realised that the only limit to what we can expect must be the number of possible interconnections that each neuron has to choose from. It is perhaps best to end this chapter in Professor Anokhin's own words:

> We can show that each of the ten billion neurons in the human brain has a possibility of connections of one with twenty eight noughts after it! If a single neuron has this quality of potential, we can hardly imagine what the whole brain can do. What it means is that the total number of possible connections in the brain, if written out, would be 1 followed by 10·5 million kilometres of noughts!
>
> No man yet exists who can use all the potential of his brain. This is why we don't accept *any* pessimistic estimates of the limits of the human brain. It is unlimited.

5 Inner Space Race

Some American ideas and an interview with astronaut Edgar Mitchell

A good deal of conjectural and wide-ranging brain research is being done in America. This is not to say that it is quantitatively or qualitatively better than in the rest of the world, but there is a perceptible bias in the work of a number of researchers. In some ways there appear to be more possibilities (or money) for a more imaginative (some might say speculative) turn of mind.

It was at SRI, the eminent Research Institute in Stanford, California, for example, that the early paraphysical experiments were conducted with the famous/infamous Uri Geller. Substantial amounts of similarly speculative work is being undertaken throughout the States, the current sensation being the research by Cleve Backster and others into the consciousness of plants. California could be called the birthplace of two-hemisphere study which is of growing importance both in terms of clinical application and philosophical discussion. Biofeedback research was pioneered in the US and many of the more tentative investigations into such elusive and controversial areas as Altered States of Consciousness are being pursued with a depth and breadth of enthusiasm less marked in other parts of the world.

An important factor, perhaps, is that America is rich and keen enough—financially and intellectually—to allow the kind of inter-disciplinary cross-fertilisation which is a fascinating aspect of modern brain research. For example, work in such disparate disciplines as those pursued by Lewis Mumford and Buckminster Fuller is seized upon as much by brain researchers as others.

The fruits of much of America's 'hard' neurophysiological research is dealt with in other parts of this book but here we may permit ourselves a glance at some of the 'softer', more speculative work. A

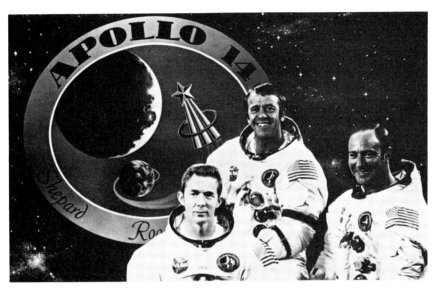

The crew of Apollo 14, Shepard, Roosa and Mitchell; Mitchell is on the right (*Space Frontiers Ltd*)

blanket term for much of this work is consciousness research: a concern with *inner space*. We quote two examples of approaches— not by neurologists as such—to solving some of our external problems; not by external means, but by using, or thinking differently about, inner space. The first is an interview with Edgar Mitchell who was the sixth man to walk on the moon. A highly qualified scientist like most of the astronauts, Mitchell established his own institute of Noetic Sciences to pursue and encourage the study of the nature of consciousness.

Q: *We usually associate the Space Programme with the summit of technology and think of astronauts as above all scientists; how is it that a highly trained man like you is working on something as allegedly unscientific as consciousness?*
MITCHELL: It's a subject that has not been addressed by the scientific community in the past, primarily because we didn't have the tools with which to really study consciousness and secondly the implications were not that important then. There were too many other

things in the world that we could investigate and solve. But scientific investigations these days, especially in physics, are recognising that consciousness is the new frontier, that we cannot go much further in physics until we start addressing these problems of consciousness. In many areas of scientific enquiry we see these lines of convergence towards the study of consciousness taking place. For me it's been a philosophic search for thirty years or more. In recent years we have started calling it consciousness but long before that looking at the inner nature of man was a passion for me. Now I think we're equipped perhaps to start doing the type of enquiry that we'd like to into the nature of man and the nature of consciousness.

Q: *You said that there were convergences and also that we now have tools to study consciousness which we didn't have before. Where else is convergence taking place and what are the tools?*
MITCHELL: Well, the most easily recognisable evidence is as I've said in particle physics, where many of the various excellent research people are beginning to get the idea that certain experiments are being defeated merely by the processes of their own minds. Now in psychological experiments, we've talked about experimental bias for several years now but even the physicists, as I say, are starting to think that in measuring subatomic particles perhaps the experimenter influences his physical experiments at these very tiny levels of force and mass and particle interaction. And many scientists are starting to say well maybe we do. There are also examples in biology. Sister M. Justice Smith, a Franciscan nun who is a biologist, has been studying the effects of so-called faith healers on enzyme systems and finding that these people called healers seem to have a track record of causing physiological changes in human beings, and can indeed affect the activity rate of enzyme systems. And enzymes seem to be very important in promoting the good health of human beings. So we see physics, biology, psychology or parapsychology, somewhat converging on the same idea that consciousness may be a fundamental key to a lot of different enigmatic problems.

Q: *What do you think of some of the new tools which are now available to us?*
MITCHELL: The most promising ones that I see on the horizon are those involving biofeedback instrumentation. Certain studies by, for

example, Dr Green, Dr Ornstein, Dr Shapiro and their associates are suggesting to us that if the individual has a measure of his physiological state whether it be by brainwaves, heartrate, blood pressure or whatever, by process of mind he is able to modify that beyond the normal limits. So I would suggest that this is a very important tool. Furthermore advanced technology, computers and all the advances in medical machinery are extending our abilities to get, as it were, on the inside in neurophysiological studies. To get inside the brain is very important; by this I mean being able to study brainwaves in great detail and so on. These are the sorts of developments that I think have a great deal of bearing on this new study of consciousness.

Q: *I know that you are studying as many aspects of consciousness as you possibly can, but I know that you do in fact have specific views yourself about what consciousness is; could you describe them to me?*

MITCHELL: First I think I must state where science currently is. I think the prevailing view certainly in psychology and in much of medicine is that consciousness results from the sophisticated computer we call the brain—in other words that it is a property of the brain. Many of the people studying this field now, however, are suggesting that this may not be the case, but that consciousness may be a totally independent quantity, equally important to the brain. In other words we don't have to think of the mind as being the same thing as the brain just as we don't have to think of consciousness as being the same thing again. Obviously they are certainly interrelated and intermeshed in a way we don't yet understand. The way I sum it up is to say that in simple terms consciousness exists and our brain is a terminal which enables us to tap into it. The very interesting, although controversial, work of Cleve Backster and his plants, which suggests that consciousness in some sense of knowing or awareness permeates down to the plant level and even perhaps down to the cellular level, is very important. Work like this is leading us to believe that these properties of consciousness or awareness are not uniquely properties of the sophisticated brain such as we humans have.

Q: *So your view is then that consciousness somehow permeates everything, but what is its source?*

MITCHELL: I wish we could say what its source is. But taking as a

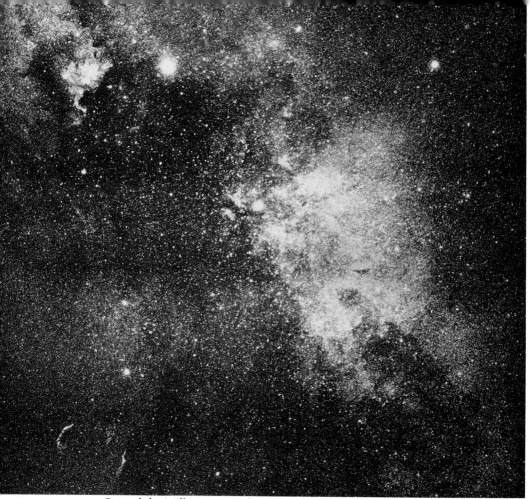

Part of the Milky Way: is there intelligence out there? (*Ross Observatory, Flagstaff, Arizona*)

working hypothesis that consciousness tends to permeate everything the next logical step would be to suggest that there is a field of consciousness that permeates the entire Universe. Field theory is popular these days in science so let us use that idea to suggest that there is a consciousness field that permeates the Universe in some way which we simply don't yet understand, and use that as a working hypothesis to start with. In this theory humans and all living systems would represent a local coalescence of a consciousness field in some sense.

Q: *You don't think that this field of consciousness is limited to our own planet. How much did your own experience in space affect your view?*

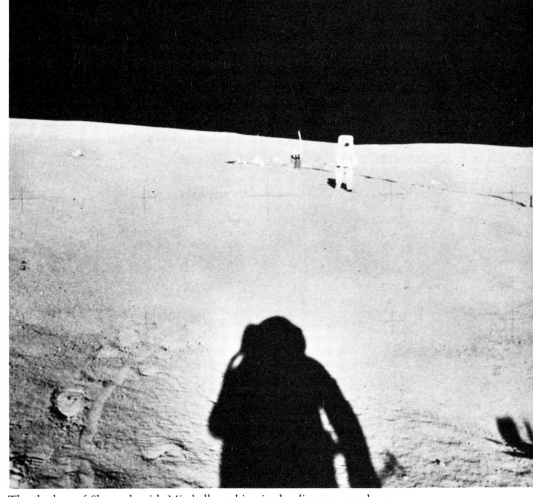

The shadow of Shepard, with Mitchell working in the distance; on the moon
each man has his own personal environment sealed into his space suit (*Spectrum
Colour Library*)

MITCHELL: Let me preface my remarks by saying that even without
any concern for consciousness or the nature of consciousness, I think
that most scientists working in any field concerned with space or
extra-terrestrial research are very well committed to the idea that
there must be other intelligence in our galaxy and certainly throughout the universe. This view is supported by statistical probability if
nothing else. The likelihood of this being a totally unique and the
only inhabited planet is almost ridiculous from a statistical point of
view. Now with that preface, my own view from space of the planet
generated several ideas. It gave me a whole new perspective of the
significance and lack of significance of the planet. When you see this

little ball of mud floating so tiny and so fragile in the universe, you recognise that it is essentially insignificant in the cosmic scheme of things. It could disappear from the universe and the universe would go right on functioning. But you recognise also that it is uniquely the birth place and home of *homo sapiens*—our own species—and in that sense it is very unique. It is our home.

Beyond that you start to recognise that Buckminster Fuller's idea that earth is like a spaceship is a very valid concept. Having travelled in spacecraft and knowing their problems one can immediately see the relevance of this analogy with the little planet earth with its finite amount of resources, its ability to sustain a very finite population, its need to be careful about environmental pollution and so on. Aboard a spacecraft we certainly must conserve our resources, we cannot dump garbage around indiscriminately, we cannot put an unlimited crew aboard, and certainly the last thing we can afford is disharmony in a spacecraft. The same things apply to earth. We have reached a stage of population, technology and sophistication in our world society where we have to start taking cognizance of the fact that our population is too big for us to sustain indefinitely at the levels of affluence we would like. Furthermore, because of our technological expertise we're ever more rapidly dwindling our sources of natural material, raw materials. The energy crisis, I believe, must surely be the beginning of a more general recognition of the shortage of resources on the planet. These are the sorts of things that came home very strongly to me as I looked at the planet from lunar distances. It is impossible not to feel a deep concern and a realisation that the problems we experience are man-made, and that man having caused these problems should certainly be able to correct them.

Q: *But why does man have to solve his problems by looking inwards into himself as it were; why can't he solve them by the normal problem-solving methods that have been used for, say, the last three hundred years?*
MITCHELL: I think we can't solve them in the traditional ways because the traditional ways have traditionally failed us. Of all the problems that we have solved, we have never yet solved the problem of getting people working together harmoniously, as brothers. Let me put it this way, as I looked back from space I became very acutely aware—

as some of our experiments are now showing—that there is a consciousness, a purpose, a divine force permeating the entire universe. We human beings seem to be in large measure oblivious to that. We seem to go about our daily lives, locked in our ethical and moral systems, each insisting on our own righteousness and fighting each other about those very issues. To me this is antithetical to the way of thinking that we're talking about in consciousness research. Furthermore, it is antithetical to survival. We cannot indefinitely continue to fight each other and waste our resources in warfare if this planet is going to survive. I think that our history has shown that the way we have thought and done business in the past will not suffice for the future. We need a new look at ourselves. Perhaps the research into the nature of consciousness, into the fundamental nature of man, using the tools of modern technology and many of the ideas that come out of the ancient past and all our religious and philosophic traditions, can be brought together in a way that will provide us with a new understanding of ourselves.

Q: *I know you feel that the power of a lot of minds working together, so to speak, has a force for the good. You quote an example of that from one of the Apollo flights, can you describe it to me?*
MITCHELL: Yes, you are referring to the Apollo 13 flight, in which the crew faced an ultimate disaster. I think it is interesting to point out that this particular mishap was one that had never been planned for. We had not trained for it because it seemed so catastrophic that most people felt: why train for certain death when there is no way to cope with that problem?

Q: *What was the problem?*
MITCHELL: The problem was the explosion of a hydrogen tank and an oxygen tank back in the service module of the command ship. Of course, when it happened, the entire team rose to the occasion and took the immediate steps necessary to save life. By applying all of their techniques and all of their knowledge the team eventually got into a situation where we thought we might just be able to get the crew back. Now without in any way suggesting that the technological expertise was not a determining factor, I will also say that I am sure that the goodwill, the love, the hope, the prayers of people around the world contributed immensely to the well-being of that crew and

their safe return to earth. From my own experimental work and from the work of many colleagues I no longer have any doubts about the power of such positive thought processes. They do affect living systems and they do affect the environment and whether we could ever prove it on such a grand scale I don't know, but in my own mind I am very convinced of it.

Q: *You are now engaged in what could be called paraphysical research and you use your prestige and influence to encourage others. Do you really think it all fits into a pattern or should the study continue simply to try and explain the so-far inexplicable?*
MITCHELL: I think that the so-called paraphysical and parapsychological studies are suggesting to us an insight into human functioning, into consciousness that we have not adequately examined before. It tells us several things. First the fact that human minds can gain information from the environment or from each other in ways that are non-sensory as we understand sensory. Secondly, it tells us that minds can influence physical matter in ways that we simply cannot explain in modern science. From this it follows that there is something about the mind and the nature of consciousness that we don't understand; beyond that it suggests that there is something about the nature of energy, matter and time that we don't understand. Certainly if the mind or some mechanism of the mind is able to influence physical matter, then there is an interaction going on here that science should look at because it suggests that the nature of matter is just not like we thought it was. Given the sort of pre-cognition studies that have been shown time and time again to produce good results, we must begin to assume that the nature of time is not as we normally think of it. So if you take all the evidence of the paraphysical and the parapsychological together it causes us of necessity to re-examine the total structure of science that has been built up over the last few hundred years. I am not saying it's wrong but I am saying that it's incomplete in some way.

Q: *But if we look forward a few hundred years instead of back, what significance do you think such work will have for human potential and man's possible organisation of himself in the future?*
MITCHELL: I would like to think that we will evolve a society in the future where mankind, individually, starts to be concerned about all

of his fellows in the same way that he is presently concerned about his family and his loved ones, where man starts to become concerned about the planet in the same way that he's now concerned about his home and his personal possessions. To me that's the beginning of it. I don't know what sort of governmental institution will evolve but I'm reasonably confident that if we can get individuals through an expansion of awareness, through understanding of consciousness, to reach out to mankind and to the planet as a whole, then the sort of institutional forms necessary to govern that sort of society will evolve naturally and it's very hard to predict what they might be. For me the first step that we have to take is for individuals to become more aware, more expansive in their thinking.

Edgar Mitchell has worked with researchers at SRI and this notable think-tank's Center for the Study of Social Policy recently devoted a great deal of resources to the production of a 347-page report called *Changing Images of Man*. The report seeks to put a new historical perspective on Man's view of himself on the assumption that there is an urgent need to modify that view to cope with this changing world in which we find ourselves. This is how they summarised their findings:

Images of humankind which are dominant in a culture are of fundamental importance because they underlie the ways in which the society shapes its institutions, educates its young, and goes about whatever it perceives its business to be. Changes in these images are of particular importance at the present time because our industrial society may be on the threshold of a transformation as profound as that which came to Europe when the Medieval Age gave way to the rise of science and the Industrial Revolution.

The recent industrial-state era can be typified by a number of almost certainly obsolescent premises, such as:

That progress is synonomous with economic growth and increasing consumption.

That mankind is separate from nature, and that it is the human destiny to conquer nature.

That economic efficiency and scientific reductionism are the most trustworthy approaches to the fulfilment of the goals of humanity.

Such premises were very appropriate for the transition from a world made up of low-technology agrarian endeavours and city-states to one dominated by high-technology nation-states; they helped to provide a seemingly ideal way to increase man's standard of living and to bring the problems of physical survival under control.

But their successful realisation has resulted in an interconnected set of urgent social problems which likely cannot be resolved through continued use of those premises; they now appear to be ill-suited for the further transition to a planetary society that would distribute its affluence equitably, regulate itself humanely, and embody appropriate images for the further future.

In contrast to such 'technological extrapolationist' future, we envisage an 'evolutionary transformation' for society as a more hopeful possibility.

Characteristics needed in an adequate image of mankind for the post-industrial future are derived by noting the direction in which premises underlying the industrial present would have to change in order to bring about a more 'workable' society; by examining the ways in which images of humankind have shaped societies in the past; and by observing some significant new directions in scientific research. A future image of man meeting these conditions would:

1. Entail an *ecological ethic*, emphasising the total community of life-in-nature and the oneness of the human race.
2. Entail a *self-realisation ethic*, placing the highest value on development of selfhood and declaring that an appropriate function of all social institutions is the fostering of human development.
3. Be *multi-levelled, multi-faceted* and *integrative*, suiting various culture and personality types.
4. Involve *balancing* and *co-ordination of satisfactions* along many dimensions rather than maximising concerns along one narrowly defined dimension (eg economic).
5. Convey a *holistic sense* of perspective or understanding of life.
6. Be *experimental, open-ended,* and *evolutionary*.

The framework demonstrates that it is at least conceptually feasible to fulfil these characteristics. Further, specific steps can feasibly be undertaken through which the fulfilment of the needed characteristics might be stimulated.

By comparing the conclusions drawn by investigators in such fields as mythology, anthropology, history of science, psychotherapy and creativity, a number of stages in a seemingly universal 'cycle of transformation' can be presented to help formulate the appropriate next steps. And by comparing the conditions of the present era with the era in which the sciences of the 'external' world were born and applied, it is concluded that a 'new Copernican revolution' may be at hand in which the birth of a new science of the 'internal' world—of consciousness and appreciation of ecological systems—is now feasible. If its development integrates appropriate methods from the arts and the humanities, it could help mankind to discover the imagery and actions necessary to raise its level of consciousness. Humanity might hereby take a next step in its evolution and hence be able to resolve many of the urgent problems of society which currently seem out of control.

While actions and policies in keeping with the 'technological extrapolationist' image would involve no great wrenching in the near term, they could lead to catastrophe or 'friendly fascism' in the longer term. Actions and policies in keeping with an 'evolutionary transformationalist' image, on the other hand, might increase the level of seeming disorder and chaos during a transition period in the near term but later lead to a more desirable society. While the choice is not necessarily one that our society as a whole will or should make consciously and deliberately at this time, it is one that confronts each individual who is willing to accept responsibility for the future—rather than simply adapt to whatever the future may bring.

Winston Churchill said: 'We shape our buildings and then our buildings shape us'. Similarly, but in a larger and more pervasive sense, we are being irrevocably shaped by our unprecedented urban-industrial environment which is premised upon images of humankind whose historical origins are far removed from contemporary reality.

The decision to supress image change or to allow social transformation confronts us with an important 'branch point' in our history. The consequences of our decisions in the next few decades will endure long into the future.

Human beings can become adapted to almost anything and since our physical and psychological endowments give us a wide range of adaptive personalities, it is crucial to distinguish between those images that foster a short term *tolerable* living environment and those that foster a long term *desirable* living environment. The dynamic character of adaptability is illustrated by a laboratory demonstration in which a frog was placed in a beaker of boiling water and immediately jumped out; when the frog was placed in a beaker of cold water that was slowly warmed to boiling temperature, however, the temperature change was gradual and the frog adapted in increments, making no attempt to escape, until he finally died. Analagously, the mere fact that a society can generate an image of the human and, for a term, adapt to it does not necessarily ensure that it would be a desirable thing to do. We can make errors and inadvertently accept images which may prove lethal both to our existence as beings seeking to unfold our potentials, and to our physical existence as an evolving species. Given our capacity to adapt—even to the point of virtual self-destruction—it is difficult to know whether or not we have already gone too far with our industrial images. Given the apparent momentum of the industrial dynamic, it is difficult to know whether we could turn back even if it seemed we had gone too far.

Nonetheless, we are still confronted with the existential choice: '. . . in matters of life . . . it does not matter whether the chance for cure is 51% or 5%. Life is precarious and unpredictable, and the only way to live is to make every effort to save it as long as there is a possibility of doing so' (Erich Fromm). We can either involve ourselves in the recreative self and social discovery of an image of humankind appropriate for our future, with attendant social and personal consequences, or we can choose to make no choice and instead adapt to whatever fate, and the choice of others, brings along.

E.B.—F

6 East-West Connections

Mysticism and technology meet

East met West dramatically when the Indian yogi Swami Rama visited Alyce Green, Elmer Green and Dale Walters, at the research department of the Menninger Foundation in Topeka, Kansas, in March 1970.

The Greens and Walters were doing some exploratory work in the field of one of man's oldest dreams: the control of his body with his mind. The Swami Rama was renowned for his ability to accomplish such feats, and consequently an experimental session at the Menninger Foundation was arranged. On his first visit, the Swami Rama was 'wired' for brain waves, respiration, skin potential, skin resistance, heart behaviour, blood flow in the hands, and temperature. While the Swami was thus 'wired' he caused two areas a couple of inches apart on the palm of his right hand to gradually change temperature in *opposite* directions. The rate of the Swami's temperature change was about 4°F per minute, until they showed a temperature difference of about 10°F. After this performance the left side of his palm, which was totally motionless, looked as if it had been slapped with a ruler a few times. It was rosy red. The right side of his hand, conversely, had turned an ashen grey. Also during this first experimental session, the Swami Rama demonstrated the speeding up and slowing down of his heart rate.

Continuing the experiments with the heart, the Swami Rama demonstrated that he could 'stop his heart' from pumping blood around his body. The Greens and Walters had assumed that his heart would actually stop beating. What happened instead was that his heart began to fire at its maximum rate, which is about 300 beats a minute, without blood either filling the chambers properly or the valves working properly. The Swami later explained that there are two ways of stopping the blood from flowing around the body. The

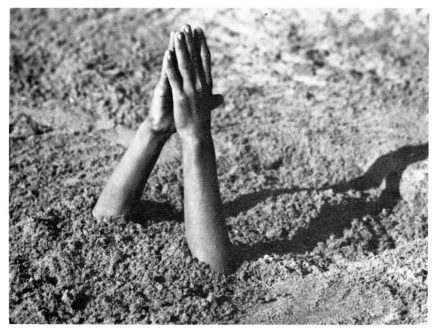

An Indian fakir buried alive (*Spectrum Colour Library*)

first, as he had demonstrated, was to make the heart 'flutter' preventing blood flow, and the second method was to go into a state of semi-hibernation in which the heart, for a brief period of time, actually did stop.

The impact of these experiments was obviously considerable, and within a few months the Menninger Foundation had published the following statement:

Aside from supporting the psycho-physiological theory previously discussed, the experiment more importantly gives us additional reason to believe that training programmes are feasible for the establishment and maintenance of psychosomatic health. If every young student *knew* by the time he finished his first biology class in grade school [secondary school], that the body responds to self-generated psychological inputs, that blood flow and heart behaviour, as well as a host of other body processes, can be influenced at will, it would change prevailing ideas about both physical and mental health. It would then be

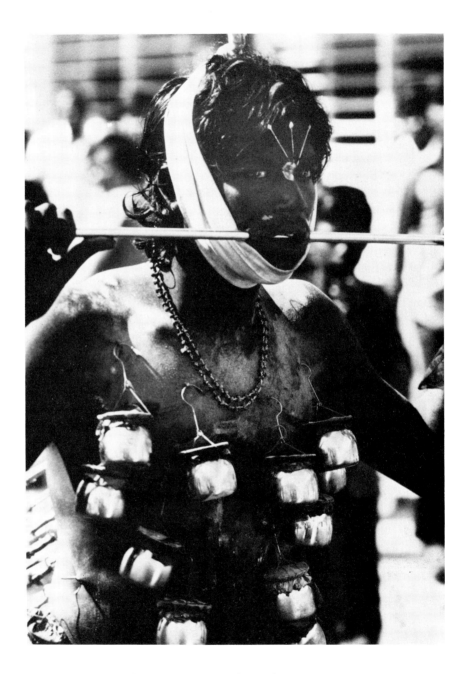

A Thaipusan in Malaysia (*Spectrum Colour Library*)

quite clear and understandable that we are individually responsible to a large extent for our state of health or disease.

Perhaps people would begin then to realise that it is not life
that kills us, rather it is our reaction to it; this reaction can be to
a significant extent self-chosen.

The final series of experiments completed with the Swami Rama
concerned his ability to control the different kinds of brain waves.
These brain waves are of four types: Beta waves, which are the waves
given off by the mind during normal attentive consciousness; Alpha
waves, which are produced when the mind is in a state of meditative
and restful awareness; Theta waves, which are produced in a near
sleep state; and Delta waves, which are not normally present except
in deep sleep.

In successive attempts, the Swami produced 70% Alpha waves over
a five-minute period of time by thinking of an empty blue sky with a
small white cloud sometimes coming by, 75% Theta waves in another
five-minute period by stilling his conscious mind and bringing
forward his unconscious, and most significantly he produced Delta
waves, sleep waves, for a period of twenty-five minutes while he was
awake! During this experiment the experimenters spoke to the
Swami every five minutes, and to their surprise found that after the
experiment in which he had produced the sleep waves he was able to
repeat the sentences that they had spoken to him, in fact with better
memory of what had been said than other experimenters who had
not known the sentences were going to be spoken, and who had been
'awake' during the experiment.

It was suggested that most people let their brains go to sleep while
their minds are still busy worrying over various matters, with the
result that they 'wake up' tired. It was again suggested that it is
necessary for the mind and brain to sleep at the same time. In the
Delta-wave state that the Swami had produced he had told his mind
to be quiet, not respond to anything, but to record everything, to
remain in a deep state of tranquillity until he actually activated it. This
state of mind was compared to that of a sleeping dog, because a dog
can leap up from a sound sleep and chase after something without
any apparent signs of having to 're-activate' itself, a very Zen-like
condition.

The researchers at the Menninger Foundation have also investigated the existence of a relationship between Theta brain waves, produced during a subjective state that they call 'reverie', and hypnagogic imagery. The Foundation was attempting to investigate the relationship between reverie, hypnagogic imagery and creativity, as revealed by many of the reports in the literature of 'intuitive' creative ideas that have come out of states of reverie and near dream. Perhaps one of the most famous examples of this kind of relationship is the story told of the chemist Kekule, who was especially able to use the creative image making facilities of his mind.

At a dinner given in his honour, Kekule told of the series of dream-like reveries in which atoms 'gambolled' before his eyes, leading to the development of his theory of molecular constitution. The last of the reveries led to his most famous discovery, which Arthur Koestler has called 'the most brilliant piece of prediction to be found in the whole range of organic chemistry'. Kekule told of growing weary while working late one night on the writing of a textbook; he continued:

> I turned my chair to the fire and dozed. Again the atoms were gambolling before my eyes. This time the smaller groups kept modestly in the background. My mental eye, rendered more acute by repeated visions of this kind, could now distinguish larger structures, in manifold conformation; long rows, sometimes more closely fitted together, all turning and twisting in snake-like motion. But look! What was that? One of the snakes had seized hold of its own tail, and the form whirled mockingly before my eyes. As if by a flash of lightning I awoke.

Kekule spent the remainder of the night working out the theory from the imagery, the structure of the benzene ring from the ancient symbol of the snake biting its own tail. It is small wonder that he urged his contemporaries 'Let us learn to dream, gentlemen.'

The results of the Foundation's experiments were most encouraging. Although there were individual differences, and although results did fluctuate from time to time, nearly all subjects were able to consciously increase Alpha and Theta production. What was more significant was that the subjects reported an increase in hypnagogic imagery as Alpha and Theta waves progressed, and also reported an unexpected number of self-integrated experiences. These experiences included increased creativity and productivity, general feelings of well being, improvements in social relationships, and an increase in both mental and physical health.

It is perhaps appropriate to leave the final word on the Menninger Foundation experiments to the members of the Menninger team:

> It seems increasingly certain that healing and creativity are different pieces of a single picture. Both Swami Rama and Jack Schwarz, a Western Sufi whom we recently had a chance to work with, maintain that self-healing can be performed in a state of deep *reverie*. Images for giving the body instructions are manipulated in a manner very similar to that used by Assogioli for personality and transpersonal integration, as in his *Psychosynthesis*. But this 'manner' of manipulation of images is also the same as that in which we find ideas being handled creatively (by two pilot subjects) for the solution of intellectual problems.

Creativity in terms of physiological processes means then *physical healing*, physical regeneration. Creativity in emotional terms consists then of establishing, or creating, *attitude changes* through the practice of healthful emotions, that is, emotions whose neural correlates are those that establish harmony in the visceral brain or, to put it another way, emotions that establish in the visceral brain those neurological patterns whose reflection in the viscera is one that physicians approve of as stress resistant. Creativity in the mental domain involves the emergence of a new and valid *synthesis of ideas*, not by deduction, but springing by 'intuition' from unconscious sources.

The entrance or key to all these inner processes, we are beginning to believe, is a particular state of consciousness to which we have given the undifferentiated name 'reverie'. This reverie can be approached by means of Theta-brainwave training in which the gap between conscious and unconscious processes is voluntarily narrowed, and temporarily eliminated when useful. When that self-regulated reverie is established, the body can apparently be programmed at will and the instructions given will be carried out, emotional states can be dispassionately examined, accepted or rejected, or totally supplanted by others deemed more useful, and problems insoluble in the normal state of consciousness can be elegantly resolved.

Three popular commercial biofeedback instruments (*Aleph One Ltd, Cambridge*)

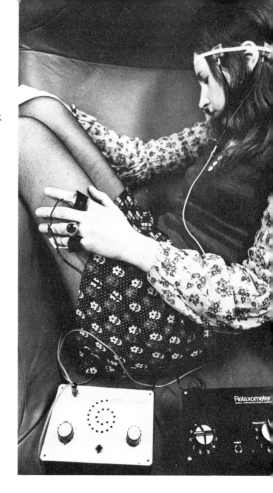

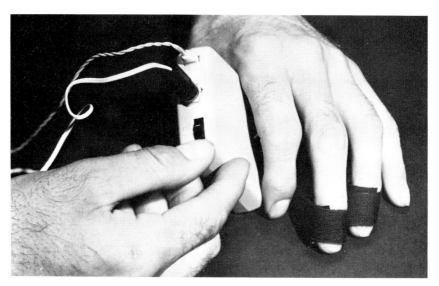

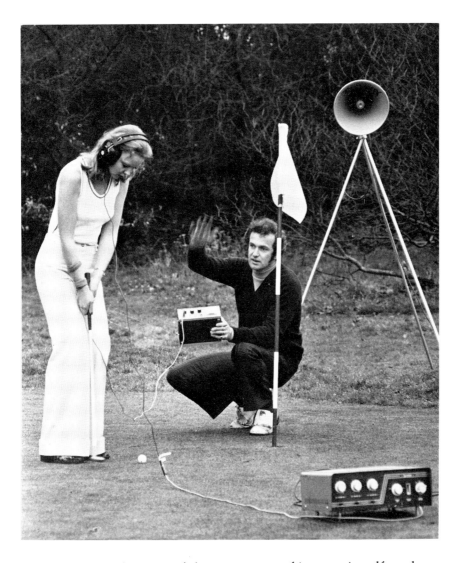

Perhaps now, because of the resurgence of interest in self-explora-
tion and in self-realisation, it will be possible to develop a synthesis
of old and new, East and West, prescience and science, using both
yoga and biofeedback training as tools for the study of consciousness.
It is also interesting to hypothesize that useful parapsychological
talents can perhaps be developed by use of these reverie-generating
processes of yoga and biofeedback. Much remains to be researched,

and applied, but there is little doubt that in the lives of many people a penetration of consciousness into previously unconscious realms (of mind and brain) is making understandable and functional much that was previously obscure and inoperable.

In the Menninger experiment, subjects were wired up to a biofeedback device which produced a certain sound when Alpha waves were being generated and another when there were Theta waves. The object of the exercise was to train the brain to be able to enter more easily into the states of consciousness associated with the generation of different waves. The Menninger work was revolutionary at the time but biofeedback is now a major growth industry in the scientific world. Two leading figures are Neal E. Miller of Rockerfeller University and Dr David Shapiro of Harvard University. Their studies have shown that individuals can control their physiological responses, and that this control can assist in the reduction of hypertension, a major disease of industrial societies, in the general healing of physical ailments, in psychiatric improvement, and in the control of mild forms of epilepsy.

Both experimenters emphasise that biofeedback techniques enable us to 'see ourselves' in a new and more encouraging light. Their findings have led them to believe that the creative potential of everyone is far greater than had been realised.

Encouragingly, individuals from the East are also beginning to apply self-analysis and the scientific method to a study of their own ability to change states of consciousness; most notable among these is the Maharishi Yogi.

There is a growing trend in brain research to attempt to integrate certain Eastern and Western ideas. One of the most significant projects in the last few years has been that concerning the two halves of the brain carried out by Professor Robert Ornstein of the Langley Porter Institute in San Franscisco. We have known for some years that the brain was divided into two halves, the left and the right hemispheres, and that the left side of our brain controlled the right side of our body, while the right side of our brain controlled the left side of our body. Professor Ornstein has recently found out that not only do the different sides of our brain control the opposite sides of our body, but that each side takes to itself certain special mental functions.

The left side of our brain, it seems, concerns itself with language, number, criticism, logic, analysis, etc. The right side of our brain is more concerned with rhythm, colour, dreams, spatial awareness, and imagination.

In his experiments Professor Ornstein 'wired up' the brains of subjects who were doing 'left hemisphere' tasks and 'right hemisphere' tasks. The EEG (electro-encephalograph) of a person taken while they were writing a letter shows that while they were writing, the lefthand side of the brain was active while the righthand side of the brain, which is not so much concerned with language, was at rest. The resulting right hemisphere was indicated by a larger proportion of Alpha waves than the left hemisphere, which showed a large proportion of Beta waves.

In the second aspect of the experiment, the subjects reconstructed abstract block designs which involved mental activity of a very different kind from that involved in writing a letter. It was noticed here that the left hemisphere was the one that produced a very large amount of Alpha rhythm, indicating that it was 'turning itself off' while the right hemisphere was producing very little Alpha and far more Beta, indicating that it was going out to do the work. Professor Ornstein has come to a number of conclusions on the basis of his work: it suggests that our whole approach to the divisions between art and science can now reach a new level of co-operation and useful understanding. In previous centuries the artist has always been divided from the scientist, despite the fact that the evidence tends to contradict this assumption. If time is taken to read the writings of the great scientists, it can often be seen that as well as producing scientific thought of enormous magnitude, they were also creative writers of considerable skill. The text books and notebooks of Newton read like the prose of the most proficient and poetic English writers.

In this debate and division, the artists and musicians have tended to come off worse. This has been because Western society has placed a greater emphasis on the scientific and analytical side of mental functioning than it has on the more colourful and imagistic side. In defence of the artists, it can be said that they have been misjudged. Once again, if the work of the artist is examined carefully it can be seen to defy the normal assumptions that it is simply 'colour placed randomly on the canvas'. The greatest artists were, upon inspection,

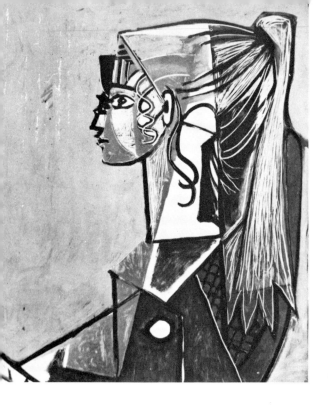

'Portrait of Sylvette' by Picasso

as close to the pure science of mathematics and physics as were the mathematicians and physicists themselves. Examine for example the works of the early masters. The nuances, shades, lines and forms were done with emotional and colourful perception, *in conjunction* with a scientific precision, accuracy and purity.

The modern movements in paintings, often maligned for being too random are, in their highest manifestations, similarly extremely scientific. The work of Picasso was *not* random shapes placed on a canvas, but was the realization of a new form of perception. For example in certain instances he was trying to indicate, on a flat plane, *all* of the different surfaces of the objects at which he was looking. The apparently jumbled shape of the Blue Lady thus becomes more 'clear'. Similarly, the work of the new visionary artist, Lorraine Gill, combines the most harmonious use of the colour spectrum with the most extraordinarily precise use of line and form. Her blending of these two elements, the artistic and scientific, produces works of art which come as close to parallelling the natural works of the universe as do the works of any artist.

The growing evidence from all these lines of research indicates some interesting conclusions. It is obvious that there *is* an East and a West, that there are artists and scientists, that the brain does have a left and a right hemisphere. But more and more the evidence suggests that if we divide, then we shall be conquered; that there is both artist and scientist in every one of us and that the more each is allowed freedom, the more each will benefit the other, producing a more complete whole. Similarly the East and the West *must* meet. Once again, the more exchange and communication that takes place, the more benefit to both and to all.

And finally, the two hemispheres of our brain must be allowed to work in harmony rather than 'living in divided houses'. All the evidence, from the work done by the Menninger Foundation, through the work done on the children with their left-right hemisphere note-taking, through the complete system theory of the leading Russians, suggests that the course is not only desirable but, in terms of the evolutionary process, inevitable.

As Ornstein himself says:
'Most of the time in our education and in our approaches towards learning about the world we have tended, if you think about it in these brain physiologic terms, to have emphasised the left hemisphere way of doing things. When we think about education we think about it as reading, writing and arithmetic, which are all the specialisations of the left hemisphere. We don't really take very seriously ideas such as art, music and dance as being aspects of education; they're usually taught in schools at least as fillers between, say, history and logic or something of that order.

'But our research indicates that our evolution has given us half of the highest level of the nervous system devoted to that other mode of thought, which I think has very great uses in a lot of different areas.

'Take an example; now a man like Einstein was *not* a man who had an extraordinarily highly developed intellect. He was not a great scholar—he failed mathematics at high school. He was almost thrown out of the college that he was in for various reasons. What he *was* extraordinarily good at was getting an intuitive picture of the universe and then having a good enough intellect to be able to translate that all-at-once picture—that sort of almost spatial insight of how things are—into the sequential and logical terms of science. And his break-through really was not our classic idea of what science is about—of little men reading these little dials and saying, 'Ah, this doesn't work' and 'That doesn't work' and 'We'll do this experiment' and so on. Einstein didn't do that at all. He just thought about the problem, was able intuitively to grasp the solution, and then was good enough to come back—so he could work in what I would call a 'complementary' manner.

'Also, if you think about what meditation exercises are designed to do, the first thing that they say is, you have to turn off your mind. What they are in essence saying is that this is an exercise which is designed to give you the opportunity to selectively turn off the normal way in which you have been approaching the world, which for us is a left hemispherish way, and begin to enter another kind of consciousness. This is a technique for temporarily disengaging the left hemisphere.

'I think it is quite important to know that many of the solutions to the kinds of problems that western science is beginning to encounter in physics, in psychology, in many areas, have been in some senses met by men of other cultures who have developed a very different mode of organising the world. By those, I mean the people of the Middle and Far East who have, if you think about it, generally had a culture organised around a more right hemispheric sense of what's important.

'It's not an either/or question that we're good and they're bad, or we're bad and they're good. But we can see the excesses of, say, our cultures as being partly because of the left hemisphere domination, of the way in which we think, what we think good thought is—and even what we think thought is. That is, when we say that someone has a great mind, we really mean that they have a great mouth—that they can speak well, that they have a good left hemisphere. We have completely rejected and almost put away that other half. You also have the counter example of people who may have extraordinarily highly developed intuitive appreciations of music and spatial awareness and the nature of reality, if you like to use those terms, who aren't linearly enough organised to clothe and feed their own cultures. So you have these great men thinking these great thoughts while people die in the streets.'

7 The Swift Idiot?

The computer and the brain
by John McNulty

Man is unique in this particular corner of the universe and he had a special role to fulfil in the process of creation. One of his new inventions has coincided remarkably with his comparatively recent discovery of his own mental processes. The computer is a novel companion, for it can be made to mimic or shadow at least some of our mentation or behaviour. It may well be that at some point we will be able to create a sentient system but until that day the computer can at least act as a very interesting mirror. Not as interesting as our children and fellow creatures but perhaps more amenable to analysis and close study without their complete destruction.

The issues we are considering when talking about the brain and the computer are severely demanding. In order to begin to understand either the workings of the brain or to create a suitable mimic of the human central nervous system with a computer, we have to alter our way of thinking. We have to try to comprehend the total working of the brain as a system, because concentration on the individual working parts of that brain will not tell us enough about the whole. Similarly, with the computer—if we wish to 'ape' intelligent man— we have to build a model which reflects the overall system characteristics of the human brain. This is not an appeal to a kind of primitive holism, but simply a restructuring of our way of dealing with the problems of intelligence and consciousness.

It is difficult to re-think one's attitudes when the change required is so alien and fundamental to our belief structures as they exist at present. Our politics to a certain degree mimic our ideas about how 'the brain' and 'the world' and 'the universe' behave. If we are to question the central issue in all our philosophies (ie the brain) then naturally we must alter our approach to all mental processes.

Without trying to promote a universal panacea, one must consider that it is most likely that the laws of organisation and structure which apply to all cellular creatures are similarly applicable to the multi-cellular organisation of our brains. It is also highly probable that the same general laws apply equally to any collection of connected individual cells, whether these cells are human biological cells or components of a computer or a society.

It has been commonly held that the structures within society or the brain follow a pyramidal organisation; that is, somebody at the top directs things, and at the bottom a large number of 'effectors' or 'workers' or even 'slaves' carry out the commands issued from the peak of the hierarchy. This belief is contained in virtually every political and philosophical model of brain or society regardless of its claims towards radical thinking. In the basic pyramidal structure which is widely assumed to exist, improvements are usually ones where the size of the pyramid is either increased or its proportions altered somewhat. It is an extremely simple model which is perhaps why it has been so popular in the past, but so is the model of the earth as a flat structure or as part of a geocentric universe.

The popular pyramid model of organisation probably springs from a picture of organisation as reminiscent of a 'tree' structure. A 'tree' model is frequently taken as being a central point corresponding to the trunk with a large number of connected sub-points corresponding to the branches. Unfortunately the analogy omits to recognise the real structure of real trees. A tree has as many root hairs as it has twigs supporting leaves. When examining a tree, one has to imagine an equivalent structure hidden from our eyes, beneath the earth, where many other branch equivalents run out into the soil. Nor is there a clearly definable recognisable organising centre in a tree; its

An artist's impression of the neurons within a human brain (Reprinted by permission of the publisher from Mussen/Rosenzeig et al: *Psychology: An Introduction*, Lexington, Mass, D. C. Heath & Company 1977.

Meditation: biofeedback experiments have demonstrated that to some extent our physiological processes can be altered at will

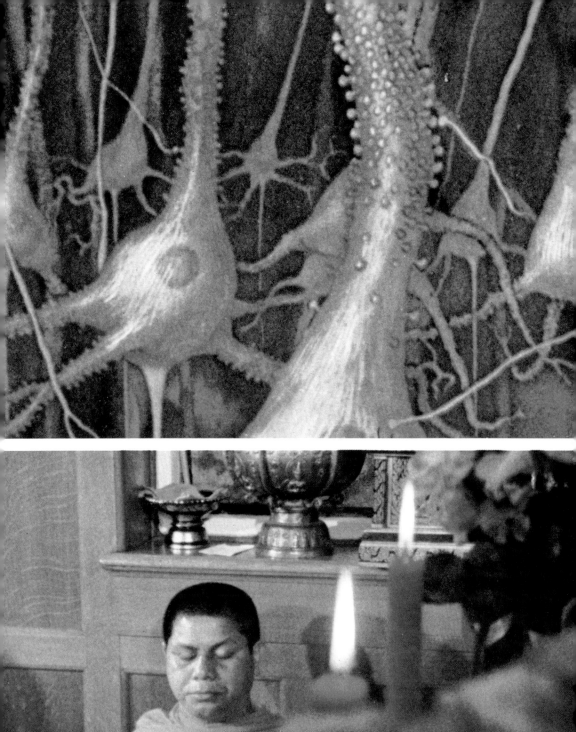

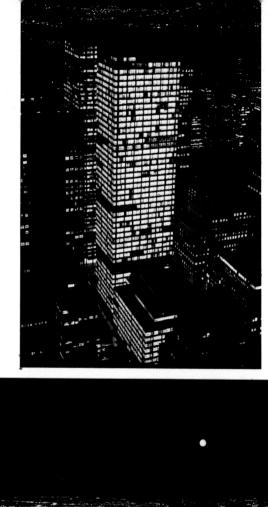
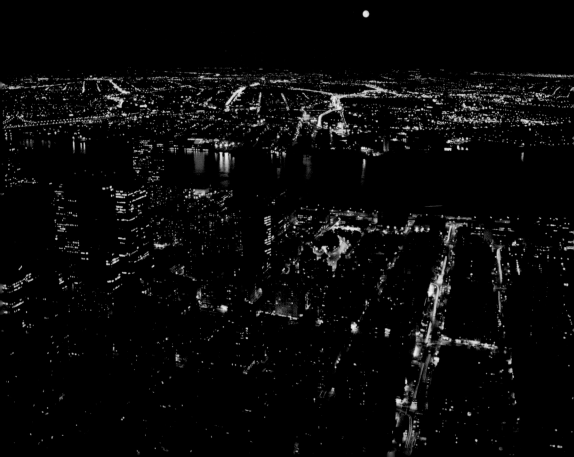

topmost bud is as much 'in charge' of the tree as the main trunk or a hair root beneath the earth. The tree, of course, is composed of many single cells, each with different and sometimes interchangeable roles. The essential idea to grasp about a tree is that it *is* and it *exists* by courtesy of the full orchestrated concert of all its cells acting together to sustain and continue life. When we begin to realise this more fully, we may well have the means at our disposal for creating a truly useful brain/computer comparison.

One usually thinks of the computer as an adding machine. It is not; it is basically a switching device—a very fast switching device. In fact a computer is masses of switches, millions of them all being switched on and off very quickly under programme control. The fact that it happens to add up as well is a little trick that we've built in— perhaps one of the most useful applications at present—but not the only one.

Generally speaking a digital computer switches between 'on' and 'off'. It operates in binary mode, which means it operates in 'yes's' or 'no's', or 'ones' and 'zeros'. When we look at the brain, we see that it too is basically a series of switches, though more complex. We need not have a direct 'on' or 'off' switch: we can have what are called 'analogue' states, for example.

In terms of speed, computers are now operating in nanoseconds and even picoseconds (a nanosecond is one thousand millionth of a second; a picosecond is one million millionth of a second). As far as we can establish the brain doesn't operate quite that quickly! It's an arguable point because one could say that at the very lowest level the electrons within the molecular tissue in the brain are being switched at those kinds of speeds.

When a human being starts thinking, the neurons are following multiple choice pathways. Each path has millions of possible

A tower block at night (above) and New York from the Empire State Building. Only at night is the random element of an organic structure like a building or a city apparent; in daylight they appear to be lifeless linear structures (*Picturepoint*)

E.B.—G

branches going off and he is making millions of possible associations and cancelling others. The indications are that while you are actually talking, you are also stacking what you have to communicate in a sort of temporary store, so that it comes out in sequence—your brain is ferreting around looking for possible associations with the next subject that you might be about to discuss.

When a person thinks in a creative manner, it is almost as though he is in a space capsule which can go in any direction: he can go down familiar ways, or he can go off on completely new ways if he chooses to. You can imagine this switching as multi-dimensional: it's almost beyond our own physical dimensional world because we're dealing with time as well. When we do something familiar we 'go through' the same mental loop or pathway. There are indications that people who become mentally disturbed (I hesitate to use that questionable classification, but the term will serve) can lapse into compulsive behaviour. Compulsive behaviour may mean that they

A large-capacity telephone exchange (*The Post Office*)

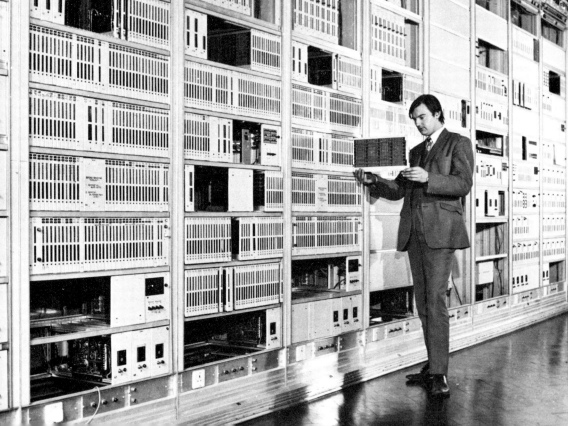

will go through a particular pathway of switches, they will go through a particular loop of behaviour time and time again, without breaking free of it. It is likely that we have many of these loops running independently all the time, probably saying things like 'is the heart running correctly?', 'is my breathing working satisfactorily?' and so on.

When we look at the recordings of brainwaves on an EEG, we can see it represents the clocking of individual rhythms or little loops which are interrogating different cells, switching around and checking that everything is all right.

We can think about a telephone exchange as essentially a very stupid brain. At present you dial the number: the connection is made slowly, and in fact we can see the actual switching taking place—we dial one and it goes switch, one, we dial five and it goes click, click, click, click, click, five, and so on. A little pathway is being traced out until we get the person at the other end and we can have a conversation. At the end we ring off and it is finished; that is like a reflex level of the brain. The next development in telephone exchanges will be to have them computer-controlled and then they will 'remember' where each subscriber is. For example: somebody rings you up, the switches fall into place finding the right route to get to you: it looks for you at your usual number, and if you are not there it goes back to its memory and indicates where you are likely to be. It can find you wherever you are, assuming of course that you want it to.

With the brain we seem to be doing exactly the same thing—we are routing automatically. When we think of something original we have to find a new routing system. Imagine an intelligent wire snaking its way round inside the brain and making multiple connections—that is what is happening.

In practice this is a poor analogy: when we talk about those 10^{10} neurons which make up the brain, we are talking about ten billion individual cells which are self-organising. They have their own identity and they are living in a kind of co-operative harmony. Each individual cell is capable of making tens of thousands of possible connections, and while it does not make all of them at the same time it has that potential throughout its life. When we think, we seem to be following certain pathways which may be very familiar. We are also looking at possible tracks which we have not used before. That

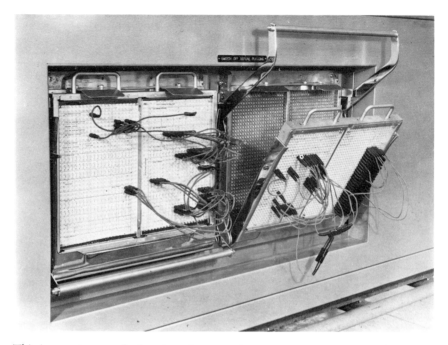

This instruction panel of an 80-column card sorting machine shows the complexity of a group of one to one connections (*International Computers & Tabulators Ltd*)

is when we get a flash of intuition, a spark of brilliance: we make a new bridge between two neurons which were not previously associated.

There are often very facile comparisons made between the brain and the computer. People fear the big bad computer taking over. Anyone who works with computers has no such fears: it is going to be a long time yet and something fundamental has to change. The computer works linearly, and though there may be many steps going on together it is still basically a linear track. When we look at the brain we have something that is working simultaneously.

A simple little device like a pocket calculator is capable of very fast calculation. This worries people: they think 'good God, what use am I, I can't add faster than that, I've only got to press a button and it adds eight digit numbers together and it will multiply, it will do square roots for me'. It uses a very small electronic circuit which is

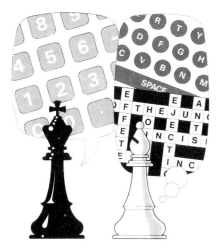

Graphic design symbolising the connection of logic, numeracy, language and chess, all logic functions of the brain which a computer may try to emulate

probably almost equivalent to parts of the brain's processing pathways.

In fact, when we add up we probably use a little more circuitry than the calculator; the brain is not designed for adding up: it is built for bigger things. Adding up is easy. Computers do repetitive tasks: they can search for masses of small pieces of information which would bore an army of clerks into the funny farm; they can switch incredibly quickly; they can control automatic processes; they can take away a lot of the boring routine that we are not interested in.

If we are going to build interesting computers—other than those that do the useful jobs, add numbers and land space craft and look after our sewage systems and so on—we are going to have to rethink our mathematics before we even begin to think about programming the computer. There's an old Bill Cosby joke that is relevant here: he is talking about his kindergarten and the teacher says '1 and 1 is 2'. He says '1 and 1 is 2: great. What's a two?' And what is a 2? What is this numerical language which we have built up? It is not real, it is simply something that we have generated for the sake of convenience. Everybody knows that this is one finger and that is five fingers, but what is it really? How many individual units are there? Can we really be accurate, can we count it down to the last possible molecule, can we count it down to the last possible molecular unit, do we know really what is in that finger when we get down to very tiny details?

There are things known as set theories and a very simple crude

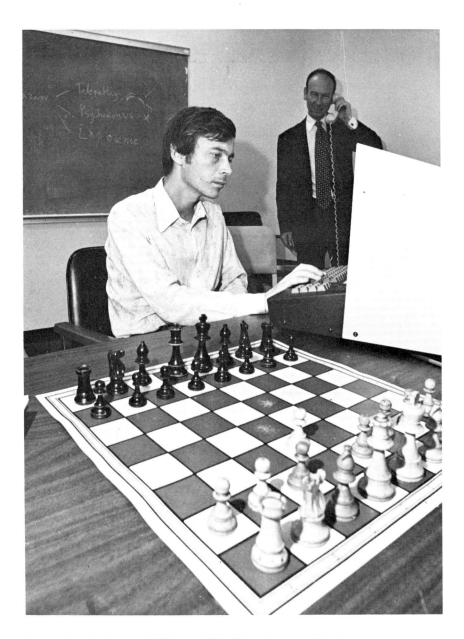

One of the developers of Kaissa, Mikhail Donskoy, waiting for a response to David Levy's opening P–Q3 move, using an Amdahl 470 V/6 computer terminal (*Computer Weekly, who run a weekly computer chess column*)

analogy of this is called Russell's paradox. This is really an extension of 'great fleas have little fleas upon their backs to bite 'em, and little fleas have lesser fleas, and so *ad infinitum*'. Russell says that no set is really big enough to totally include itself: in other words if you try to describe something numerically you also have to describe the thing that you are describing it around and you cannot bracket yourself within that description so you are constantly trying to bracket something that is too big.

The computer, however, is accurate and it has perfect recall (in theory). It is also extremely flexible if we programme it to be that way. Anybody who has had a bill for £0.000 will not agree with that, but in fact the computer can be programmed to be extremely flexible. For example, imagine a committee meeting which is having difficulty resolving the best town plan or the best airport to build: they have to take into account many factors. Although an architect can draw a very good plan, and the civil engineers can design a very good bridge structure, and so on, the amount of data that is being handled becomes too much. It is boring routine data and yet it has to be called up in cases like this where people do not have a common data base. Then it is possible for people to put alternative hypotheses to the computer. It is possible to use a dynamic model to dynamically change a picture based on much data which no single individual has.

So there is a great potential for computers as 'artificial limbs', if you like, for the brain—things to help us remember, things to help us simulate possible conditions which we could not hope to simulate physically. We could build an airport and then find out it was wrong, but it is very expensive and it takes a lot of time: with a computer we can just press a button and a new airport will appear so that we can see what the possibilities are.

The best analogy one can make in terms of people and the brain is something like a city. Look at London, with about 12 million people within the Greater London Council area. London just grew up; nobody planned it. If we look at the map of London we can see that it is a whole network of interconnections—rail routes, road routes, telephone routes—all leading in. And yet it has no actual centre. We say 'the city' or 'the centre of London' but there is no single central point: it is a massive maze which has slowly built up. It looks very similar to a section through a brain, showing blood vessels and neuronic pathways. Within that brain of London each individual is making free choices. He is saying, 'I've got friends, I want to talk to these people'; he is switching between possible connections, he is ringing people up, he is going and meeting people—and each of those individuals is acting very much like a neuron.

In fact it is probably quite valid to argue that unless we are fulfilling our role as neurons within a sort of global brain, we will not feel really satisfied. When we are dealing with people we get information coming in, we switch it to somebody else, we make choices all the time; unless we do that we begin to feel dissatisfied with life. There is evidence from stimulus deprivation experiments that unless we do make connections and unless we do have real information flowing through us—not just landing on us passively, but flowing through us and being modified by us—we feel unfulfilled.

Now we can look at the wider question of the brain and the world. There are now around three and a half billion people in the world (or three and a half billion plus 200 because another second has gone by). All these individuals can be in touch with each other: potentially any individual can contact any other individual on the earth within a very short period of time. Many of them do not, but that is irrelevant. Yet within our brain we have now at least *ten* billion neurons talking to each other; they manage our brain—a far more complex organisation than society.

When we look at the earth we are looking at the equivalent of a pretty small brain. Of course I am neglecting to point out that each of those individual units in the world is itself a brain with ten billion neurons within it, so society is in fact far more complex. But if we view people as components of neurons within that brain called society, we have only three and a half billion; the brain has got ten billion and it's pretty smart.

The key to the brain's successful organisation as opposed to society's often inefficient functioning is in the nature of the system. As was pointed out at the beginning of this chapter, we have tended to create pyramidal or linear systems. For example we can go into the head office of a large organisation and look at a wallchart to see the chairman at the top and the workers at the bottom linked by all those chains of command. Fortunately there isn't a chairman in charge of the brain; management is handled by each individual neuron, with clumps of neurons which take responsibility for a particular function (there must be clumps now that are having a look at my heart occasionally to make sure that things are all right).

There are two fundamental things wrong with the pyramidal organisation. First it is very good for passing messages *down*, but it is very bad for feedback—if the worker at the bottom wants to tell the chairman that something is wrong with the firm there are all those chains of command on the way. There is also the 'whispering game' syndrome, because each individual on that chain is going to distort the information somewhat so that by the time it has got back (if it ever gets back at all) it is hopelessly distorted and probably far too late. Of course, anybody who has worked in an organisation knows that this hierarchy does not work. The chart is useful as a reference point but without *real* structure, an infrastructure, within it the system simply does not function.

You can picture a factory where say three times a month the night watchman actually controls the running of the factory, or the receptionist and switchboard operator actually control the profitability of the firm. Nobody will notice this and their wages will not reflect it—and the individual people probably do not know it. But the control structure within that organisation may well depend on feedback and information being switched by those individuals. If the nightwatchman does not leave the doors open for the late lorries to come in and deliver their loads to the end of the assembly line, the work of the early morning shift can be disrupted without anybody in management knowing it. If the shift does not get the thing out on time, the next job is interrupted and they lose an export order—and so on. Similarly the girl on the switchboard is in a key position and yet people do not seem to realise that the way she handles information switching can often determine how sales go and how people are located.

We cannot put an 'X' on the brain and say that is the seat of consciousness, there is a seat of understanding, there is the soul. All we can say is that there is a consciousness that is shared by those billions of interacting cells and that the centres of command change and shift as the information changes. In fact you can almost view it as a sort of amoeba, an abstract amoeba. Information comes in, the amoeba of the neuronic networks changes to accommodate and engulf that information, it lets the information flow through, and it is itself changed by that information coming through.

What we have tried to do with computers is to have a boss at the top—the programmer. That is why we have limitations. The reason a good chess player can beat a computer is because we have tried to impose on the computer a rigid hierarchical structure. We may have choices within that structure but when it is reviewing possible moves it has to run through an incredible number of combinations—it is doing far more *effortful* work than our brain is. When we are playing a game of chess our brain is capable of knocking away all the irrelevant moves, whereas a computer has to seriously consider each stupid move—sacrificing the queen, or treating it as a pawn. It has to consider the possible movements of every single piece and can quickly run out of possible 'cells' within its 'brain' to deal with it because it has to look at every single linear step. Somehow the brain works by cutting out all the irrelevance all the time.

We can extend the analogy of the global world brain even further when we think about the future. Telecommunications will change the whole world in a way which as yet is only dimly understood. Returning to the theme of computers as switches, it may have occurred to you already that a telephone exchange simply consists of a great many switches. At present these switches are large and cumbersome and very slow, but if we replace the old-fashioned exchanges with the latest tiny and incredibly fast computers, amazing new possibilities occur.

We also must consider the virtual disappearance of millions of miles of cables and wires which we now take for granted. Just as the old overhead telephone lines have slowly disappeared, so in the near future will most of our underground connections fade out of use because of the emergence of the communication satellite. So far communication satellites have only influenced transoceanic calls and the relay of television programmes such as the Olympics, the Moon Shots and the Commonwealth Games. These communication satellites hold out an infinitely greater promise to the future hope and prosperity of mankind than many of us can now realise. When we start to integrate our increasingly smaller and faster computers with the communication satellites we will end up with intelligent telephone exchanges in the sky. This will dramatically reduce the cost of any individual's communication with any other individual in the world, and will make possible a volume of trade and information interchange that we cannot comprehend.

Every single facet of our lives will be altered by these exchanges in the sky. Education will develop into an exciting inter-active dialogue reminiscent of the old personal tuition but with the combined knowledge, resources and wisdom of the entire world at the student's fingertips. The intelligence of the exchanges will make it possible for us to reach any people with whom we share an interest, no matter what their location. The resources of the world will be matched more evenly with the requirements of mankind. Cities will become decongested and commuters will become ruralised as we work by wire and toil by telephone. The unique loneliness of an individual in the city will be banished and distance will truly be no object. New scientific ideas will permeate the globe and be integrated into our body of knowledge within days of their discovery. Anyone who has anything to buy or sell will be sure of an instant response. But the real change in our lives is not so easy to describe.

The picture of the world as a sort of brain with all the individuals acting as neurons—a kind of world brain—will daily become more tangible and more distinct. We cannot really imagine the awakening to full consciousness of this world brain but if we can picture the power and energy of the Renaissance multiplied a millionfold, we may be on the right track. If we imagine the development of a child's brain into the early stages of informed consciousness and multiply that awakening by approximately five billion, then we may have a faint understanding of what we will witness when the brain of our planet awakens and recognises itself for what it really is.

8 City-Brain or Brain-City?

An analogy
A personal view by Terence Dixon

Society's brain is the city. It is the nerve centre, the master control of communications, the seat of most of the higher functions and aspirations. Its libraries, museums and records are society's 'memory'. Its laws and traditions are the inherited information. Like the brain, the city must exist in symbiosis with its 'body' and obtain nourishment from it. Its waste must be removed via the 'body'. It must delegate functions. .

All this is no surprise, of course, since our brains created our cities. To some extent we have created huge extended models in the outside world of what goes on inside our own heads. The analogy has its limits, but the parallel growth of research into the brain and the city has been mutually useful. In studying both we learn more about ourselves and our needs. It is a truism that we can never fully understand our own brain, because we are using it to examine itself. The most significant fact about the brain, as we have seen in Chapter 1, is that it is far greater than the sum of its anatomical and physiological parts. To explain everything about it, to reduce its functions to something completely describable in scientific or any other terms, would imply that the author of the description had a larger analytical capacity than a brain. As the Zen masters say: 'the eye cannot see itself; the hand cannot hold itself'. We can never completely describe or quantify the city either. Each one is different and changing all the time. Each is composed of perhaps millions of individuals who also defy complete description and who are, in turn, changing all the time in themselves and thus changing their cities, day by day, minute by minute.

But, of course, we can improve. We have seen, in previous chapters,

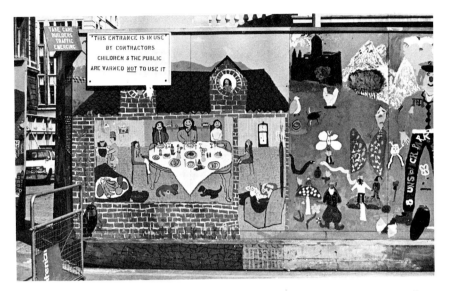

Mural showing how children have decorated part of their city (*Spectrum Colour Library*)

something of how brain research is progressing; how work all over the world is illuminating not only the brain itself but, more importantly, many areas of human activity which were previously thought —as if it were possible—to have almost nothing to do with the brain. However ultimately limited we are, the more we learn and apply what we learn about the brain the better. The brain is the most complex system in nature; the modern city the most complex social system in history. Some of the parallels between the two systems have been mentioned, others will follow. It is a metaphorical comparison, but a useful one. If we look at our cities we can learn something about our brains because they created them: if we look at our brains we should learn more about how our cities perhaps could work.

Despite a prevailing assumption in some quarters that the essence of the city is to be found in its buildings and facilities, it is important to remember that a city is really people. It is organic—a city without people is the brain of a dead man: tissue without function. Mozart's brain alone can compose no more quintets; the Houses of Parliament mean nothing without people inside. The city is organic in another sense. It must grow and develop in the same way as any other organic

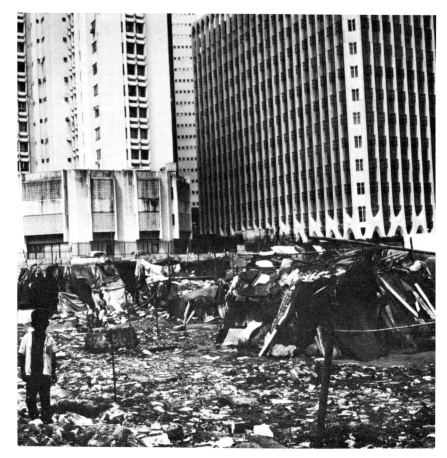

Stark contrast in Bombay, India, between poverty and new development (*Spectrum Colour Library*)

thing. Studies have been made which demonstrate that the sudden and inappropriate creation of the material structure of a modern city in an underdeveloped country is like grafting the brain of a sophisticated person onto the body of a two-year old child. Lusaka is a case in point.[1] It grew dramatically in the sixties and the 'body' could not cope with it. In 1962 Lusaka produced 30,000 tons of waste. In 1970

[1] Dr Francis Shattock, University of Liverpool, is preparing a book which includes such a study. The figures quoted are his.

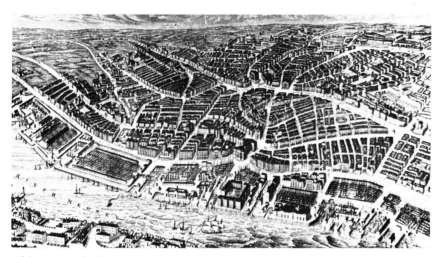

Old Liverpool – like the neurones of the brain the roads curve out from the heart of the city into the countryside

there were 150,000 tons—an increase of 500%. In 1962, 9½ million gallons of sewage was removed from the city; by 1970 they could remove only 12½ million gallons—an increase of only 30%. As well as choking itself, Lusaka is using up resources which would be better used elsewhere in the country. In 1960 it used 2½ million gallons of water a day. In 1971 it used 15½ million gallons, without growing a single crop. The physical trappings of 'modern' city administration, even the schools and hospitals, in no sense serve the real needs of the country. The country cannot afford the city. It drains precious resources required for more basic development. One man can have a complicated heart operation while thousands of children die for lack of simple hygiene. Lusaka's rapid growth is also non-evolutionary. The average annual population increase of 11·8% in the sixties was made up of 10% immigration from outside the city. These migrants are notoriously ill-adapted to live in cities. They cause themselves and the cities all too familiar problems. In Lusaka, some 50% of the population live in squatter compounds. They are the damaging 'foreign bodies' in the system. It is not fanciful to say that such a system is biologically unnatural. It is a grotesque hybrid which would never have evolved in a natural way.

This is not to say that older cities which did grow more gradually and naturally are all splendid examples of evolution triumphant. Few people would argue that London or New York, for example, are Gardens of Eden with modern sanitation, but the evolved cities do have a better developed system. And that system, to quote Professor Luria (see Chapter 4), resembles the function system of the brain.

Although the city, like the brain, has specialised areas which fulfil certain functions—seats of government, commercial centres, residential areas, etc—it is obvious that the city as a whole can adjust quite readily if something happens to disrupt the distribution pattern. Professor Luria argues that localised functions can be taken over by other areas of the brain if brain lesions occur. This is not a simple matter, especially if the damage is severe, but it can be done. In the same way, London survived as a living city, with most of its operations functioning, during the bomb damage of the Blitz. If London's 'City' area were to be destroyed tomorrow, the immediate consequences would no doubt be traumatic, but in a short time London would be continuing with its traditional role as an international financial and business centre. The physical location might be different, but it would remain part of the function system of the city.

A city is a conglomeration of people, just as a brain is an assembly of ten billion neurons. It can even be argued that people are the neurons of the city/brain (Chapter 7). We can certainly see that it is in fact the millions of interconnections between the individuals in a city that keep it going. If no-one moved, talked, telephoned, or connected with anyone else at all, London would collapse in an hour. The buildings would stand, but it would not be a city. Professor Anokhin has demonstrated (Chapter 4) that each single neuron in the brain has a virtually infinite potential for interconnection. Theoretically, as John McNulty has argued (Chapter 7), this could be true of people in the communications-rich city of the future.

Two examples of right hemisphere dominance: a highly developed sense of spatial awareness (above), but not linearly organised enough to clothe and feed their own people (below) (*Spectrum Colour Library; Picturepoint*)

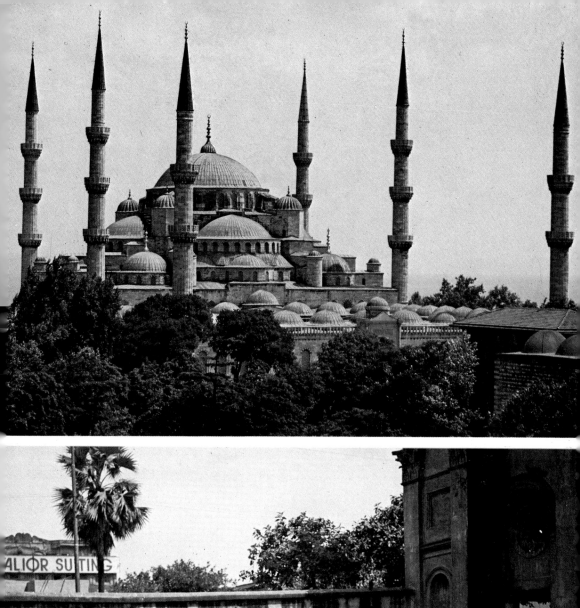
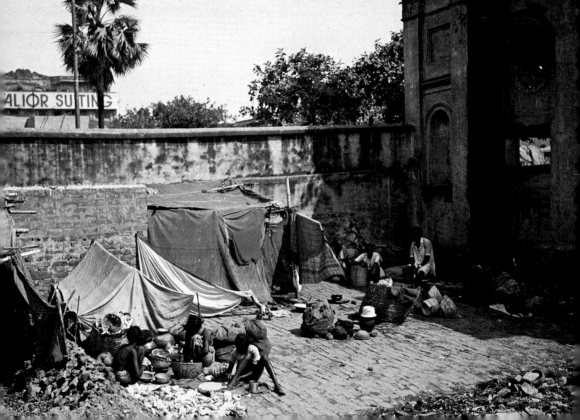

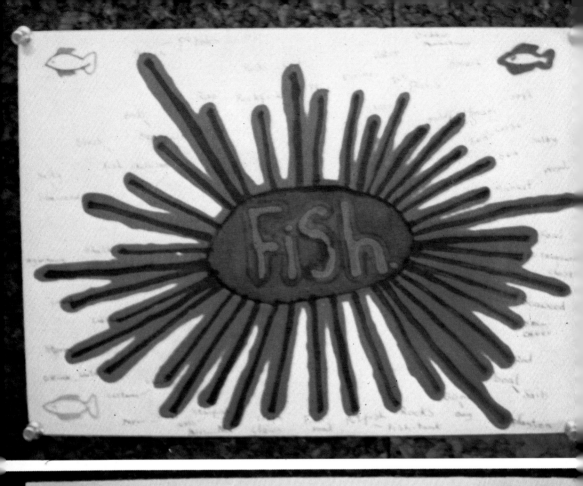

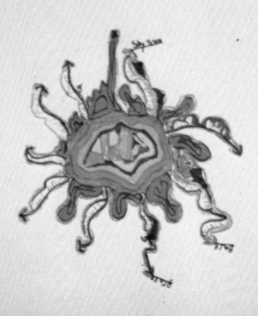

Shadrach
Chitolic

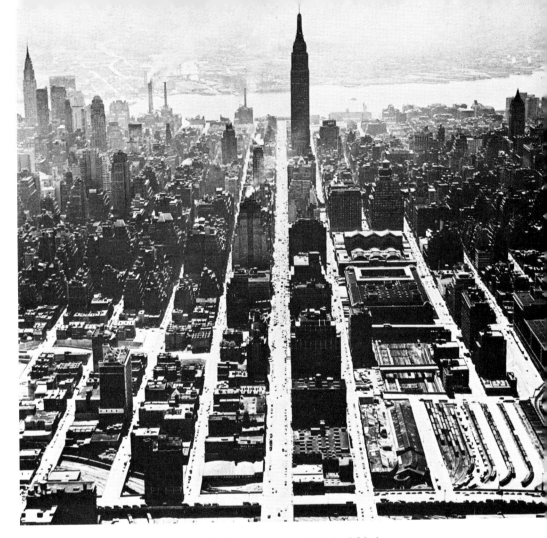

New York – straight streets in a perfect linear pattern (*Weidenfeld & Nicolson Ltd*)

Towards mind patterns: examples of children's work (see page 35)

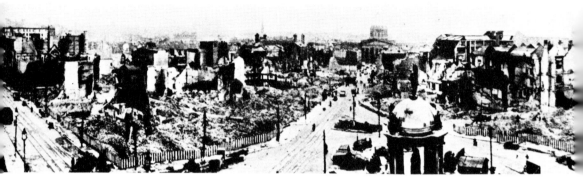

Liverpool: although destroyed in the blitz, street patterns remain

Mark Rosenzweig's work has shown that a stimulating and varied environment leads to physical growth in the number of connections among neurons in the brain (Chapter 1). In the city context we can observe this phenomenon in reverse. The citydweller with many friends, an active social and cultural life, many amusing places to go—in other words with many connections—would certainly claim that his environment was stimulating. This is, of course, part of the great strength and value of the city.

But not everyone likes the city. For some it is a place of unique and paradoxical loneliness. We can easily understand that this loneliness, this impoverished personal environment, is a lack of necessary connections. It is indeed a bitter paradox because, as we have seen, the brain—the person—demands stimulation just as forcefully as the body demands food.

The city is disliked for many other reasons. 'The concrete jungle' is a vivid and familiar term of abuse. Noise, pollution, crowding, dehumanisation and stress are all frequently quoted by back-to-nature advocates who hold that the modern city is a most unnatural place for human habitation. This is an understandable point of view, but it has a two-fold weakness. In the first place it assumes that the city has some life of its own; some self-generating mechanism from which the hand and mind of man are excluded. This is just not so. Machines do not make noise or pollute of their own volition. They are neutral objects which do not become unpleasant unless men want

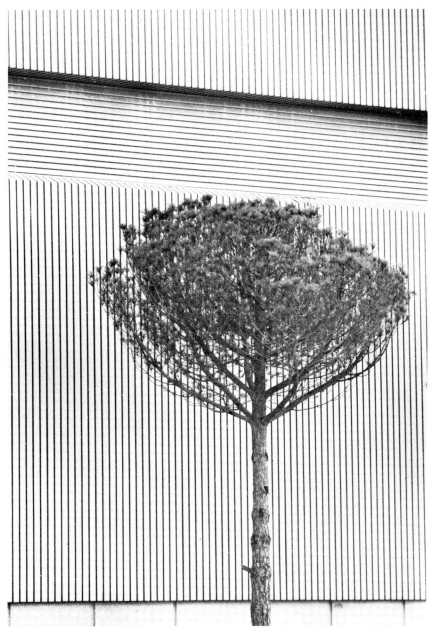

A building with a particularly linear design relieved by the placing of a natural object, a living tree (*John Chard*)

them to, or want something else so much that any ill effects are tolerated, at least by those who produce them. Secondly, the city is a completely natural thing in a complete human sense. A pre-stressed concrete house is no less natural than a mud hut. Man makes both from the earth's resources. Plastic may replace wood, steel may replace stone, but the principle is the same. The stock exchange is a *natural* extension of the tribal gathering around the cooking pot. Television is a *natural* extension of the smoke signal—even of the human voice. And so that which we may dislike about the modern city is, whether we realise it or not, simply that which we dislike about ourselves, or part of ourselves.

The split-brain analogy is obviously appropriate here (see Chapter 6). The two basic types of higher brain function do appear to reside in the two different hemispheres. It has been argued that, in our society, the concerns of the left hemisphere have been emphasised at the expense of those of the right. The swiftest glance at any modern Western city would certainly confirm the view that money is favoured by our society above beauty, that order and regularity seem more important to us than creativity and spontaneity. There is no evidence from brain research to indicate that the left hemisphere is more *important* than the right, however. In neuro-physiological terms they are of equal significance. It is simply that in our culture we use the one more and tend to neglect the other. In Chapter 6 this split-brain work was linked with the differences between what can generally be described as the Eastern and Western modes of thought. Eastern ideas and traditions can be seen to embody right-hemisphere dominance in the way that ours lay emphasis on the left. This comparison can be extended to the problems of cities as well. To a large extent the difficulties of the ancient cities of, for example, the Indian subcontinent such as Bombay and Calcutta can be seen to stem from a form of left-hemisphere deficiency. The Eastern mind is often considered illogical by the Westerner—as perhaps it is, though this need not be adverse criticism. Certainly the qualities required to organise mass production, vast housing schemes, transport networks and agricultural programmes are not as conspicuous in the East as they are in the West. Hence the horrors of those Eastern city streets. And yet there is much to admire in Eastern cities. Plumbing is not everything.

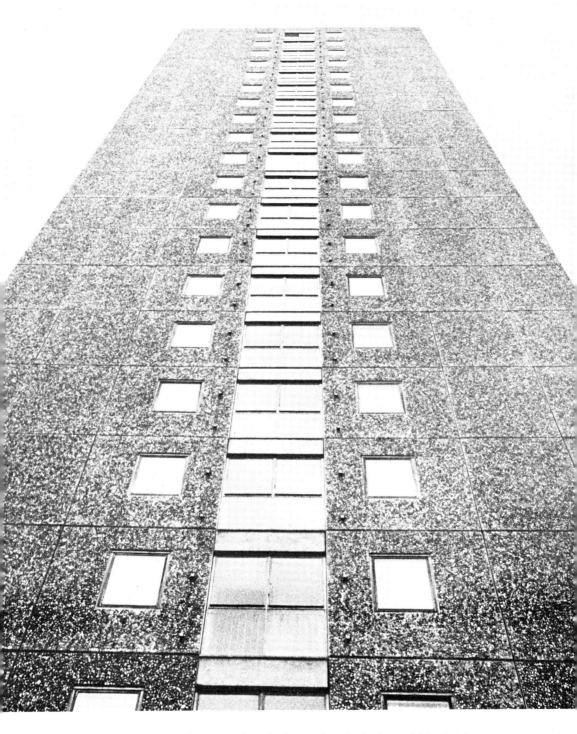

A strictly linear tower block (*Weidenfeld & Nicolson Ltd, photo: Mike St Maur Sheil*)

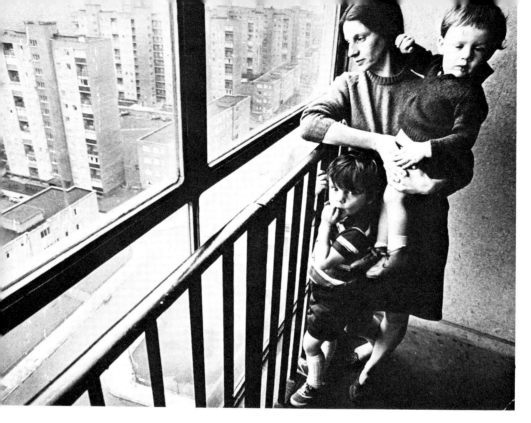

A mother and child imprisoned in their high-rise block (*Weidenfeld & Nicolson Ltd, photo: Mike St Maur Sheil*)

In our cities in the West, it does sometimes seem as though only physical requirements are considered by the planners. To run a city is not easy. Naturally enough, those in authority are those whose inclinations lie in what might be called a left-hemisphere direction. They organise, they plan, they do sums, they consider efficiency. This is linear thinking and leads to linear results in every way—in the buildings themselves and in the bureaucracies that run them.

In Chapter 7, John McNulty pointed out the limitations of linear bureaucracy in business organisations. The same is true of city councils. It can hardly be a coincidence that tower blocks resemble the organisation structure which creates them. These buildings are not designed by people for people. They are designed by people for *other* people: for people on paper—non-people.

It is hardly tolerable to work in a relentlessly linear environment—on a production line, in a routine office—even if the pay is good. But there is at least a social value in mass-producing goods cheaply, provided they are goods that we want. Anyone who denounces

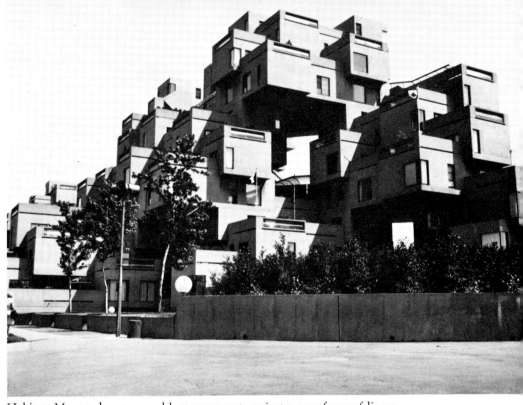

Habitat, Montreal: a new and better concept, or just a new form of linear development? (*Spectrum Colour Library*)

washing machines may never have handwashed dozens of nappies every day. But living in rigid straight lines is another matter. It is simply biologically unnatural for us to live literally on top of each other, or in long unbending rows. The natural form of social grouping is irregular clumps, so that other people with whom we can interact cluster in every direction. The brain, as we have seen, operates on a multi-dimensional basis—we know that a paperback book is not a postcard because we have seen them both before from many angles and we have learned about depth, real shape and perspective by having a constantly changing view of objects. Our brains respond best to *differences*: to variety in shape, texture, colour and all experience. Our right hemispheres—half the highest level of our nervous systems—are concerned with aesthetic, spatial, tonal considerations. In view of all this, our brains can hardly enjoy a uniform box on the twenty-fifth floor. And yet blocks like the one shown above left are supposed to support communities. They encase hundreds of multi-dimensional brains in linear conformity. The only defiance of this enforced regularity can be seen at night. Then the lighted windows meekly reveal the more random patterns of real life

It is not surprising, therefore, that many people seem to prefer the apparent irregularity of 'unspoiled' nature outside the cities. The trees appear to group as they will, the wild flowers grow in seeming confusion, the vista changes from day to day, from season to season. But, of course, nature is not really quite as haphazard as that. She has her laws, rules and demands, as the ecologists are swift to point out to us. What the citydweller may find in the countryside is a vast physical and biological system which is self-regulating, just like the physical and biological system inside his own head.

Perhaps modestly, we seem to assume that a system we create can never suit us as well as a system we did not create, which indeed may have created us. Modesty is a good Victorian virtue, but not very appropriate when applied to the seemingly infinite capacity of the brain. And the industrial city, one of our profoundest Victorian inheritances, does not seem a very appropriate place for the brain. We will never solve the problem completely, just as we can never fully comprehend the brain. But we can attempt to alleviate some of the grosser incompatabilities. If we can make the function system of our cities more similar to the function system of our brains; if we move towards a city that is less regulated and more self-regulating, we will be making progress.

This is not to suggest that we make the city more 'natural' in the naive sense of destroying material things, dismantling technology and living under trees. We are no less in tune with nature, in the widest sense, when we sleep in a warm bed as opposed to a muddy bank. Because we made the city, we can make it more habitable, more human. We must accept apparent opposites. The problem is often that we assume opposites cannot be reconciled, that two or more ways cannot all be the right way at once.

Two major dilemmas in current thinking about the city concern money and planning. In both areas the protagonists divide into opposing camps. On the one hand, it is argued, too little money is spent on providing intangible facilities for people—open space, human perspectives, a *sociable* environment—and this is certainly true. On the other hand, the argument goes, money is irrelevant to these problems: 'throwing cash at them' is no solution; concern not cash is what is required. This is also true. As for planning, one point of view is that only vast comprehensive development schemes can work. The Greater London Development Plan is a case in point. Only in this way, some say, can all the vital, interconnecting problems be solved.

The other point of view is that this is dehumanisation on an epic scale, the reduction of individuals to helpless pieces in an impersonal game of bureaucratic chess. Each of these arguments is equally valid, What is required is not resistance to, but an acceptance of, these fundamental paradoxes. The paradox seems problematical only because we are physically and temporally incapable of *saying* two things simultaneously. The brain, which can happily do countless things at once, helps us here again. It can love and hate together, it can be calculating and irrational at the same time, it can value trees and enjoy the endless newsprint which is destroying them. It has a left and a right hemisphere which only appear to oppose when one is used at the *expense* of the other.

The neurons in the brain are independent but, acting in unselfconscious concert, they do produce overall strategies. We can see, we can hear. Strategies for our cities must involve specialists—bankers, planners, politicians. But this should no more mean that any individual's needs must be ignored than the fact that I am listening to a Bach recording means that I cannot hear my baby cry at the same time.

There can be no complete solutions. Many of the problems of the past and present are the result of an assumption that there ever was such a thing as *the* correct solution. Everything changes all the time. The city needs less regulation and more self-regulation. That means accepting some paradoxes. If a little of the energy (and money) presently expended in preparing cases against equally valid propositions was used to consider all of them simultaneously and harmoniously, our lives would be transformed. If a greater understanding of ourselves, of our brains' systems, was allowed to permeate the organisation of our cities, they could become as 'natural' an environment for us as the highland air is for the golden eagle.

9 A New Renaissance?

A hopeful look ahead

The sudden explosion of 'mind information' may well be the most significant turning point in man's evolutionary history. The data now pouring from laboratories and research centres around the world has already provided us with information which allows us more easily to change our basic concepts about the nature of ourselves, our universe, and our social and cultural relationships.

The fact that our brains are divided into two hemispheres lays low many of our previous misconceptions. We now know that in each of us lies dormant the ability to express ourselves in either the artistic or the scientific mode: that the highest level of our nervous system has been apportioned equally to these two aspects, and that when each is functioning well and freely, the total output, creativity, and balance of the system is far greater than the sum of the two halves.

This area of research is still in its infant stages, yet even now further studies are indicating that the probabilities for combining 'opposite' areas of human abilities are far greater than a simple 'left/right' division. Rather than containing one possibility, it appears that each one of us may in fact contain a crowd.

The statistics uncovered by Anokhin on the phenomenal number of biochemical permutations and combinations of interconnections between the branches of our ten billion brain cells are more than mere statistics. The figures indicate that each individual is *far more* individual than had been previously realised. We now know for a fact that each human being is unique not in just a few specific characteristics, but is unique in the more than trillions of special and personalised interactions and patterns that he has experienced throughout a lifetime, and has stored in what we now know to be an increasingly voracious memory.

Underlying Anokhin's statistics was the crucial observation that each individual brain cell was both independent and interdependent. Each cell was able to make its own specific decisions, but seeming to do this always in a 'reasoned' consideration of the events affecting the person, and the decisions being made by other brain cells surrounding it. The implications on a larger scale are significant. From this basic and inherent model the reason can be found for ceasing the devisive thinking currently popular in psychology, sociology and politics. Rather than creating models in which the individual is all-important and the group insignificant, or models in which the group is paramount and the individual 'lost in the morass', a new model can be devised in which both individual and group are accepted as unique, independent yet interdependent.

In the light of these and other awarenesses concerning the complexity and potential of our minds, the often-quoted threat of the computers can be put into a realistic perspective. In comparison to our own organic meta-computers, the poor mechanical imitators of some of our basic functions can hardly be seen as threats. When it is realised that the intelligence of the most sophisticated computer is the equivalent to that of an earthworm, and that the interconnections in *one* brain are one million times greater than all the interconnections of the world's entire telephone systems, the assumed threat of the 'enemy' dissipates. Far from dehumanising us and taking away our identities the computer, if properly used, would be nothing but a force for good, taking over the more mundane of our mental functions, and thus leaving us free to explore other areas.

Any information on our minds will have, and is already having, profound effect on our approach to education. Realising the extraordinary flexibility of our central nervous system, we now have little choice but to change the way in which we approach our early nurturing and training of it. Each child can now be seen as a beautiful potential, a highly sensitive being containing almost unlimited possibilities. When faced with a being far more sensitive than a million-filimented anemone, one whom one wrong word can send into an instant and total withdrawal, our responsibilities automatically become enormous.

To begin with, our antiquated approaches to testing will have to change. To date we have been educating our children to think in linear, restricted manners, testing them on that basis and then expressing surprise that they scored poorly and seem to exhibit 'basic' inflexibility and rigidity; what we have been doing of course, is creating a situation, measuring it, and then assuming that that situation 'naturally' exists. Nothing could be further from the truth.

Recent experiments based on the new information concerning the potential of the brain have already shown that basic IQ and creativity tests can be consistently 'broken' once the child knows the proper functioning of his mind. Hundreds of individuals have gone from mediocre and poor average scores to off-the-top-of-the-scale scores after being given the 'key' to their functioning. Testing in the future will probably be used as a measure of lack-of-training rather than a measure of 'inherent natural ability'.

Similarly our approach to order and freedom within the classroom will change. We have often confused order with rigidity, and freedom with chaos. Rather than having classrooms specifically regimented in terms of subject matter and time, or classrooms in which everything is random in order to foster 'creativity', classrooms will combine a basic organisational structure, with a freedom for the individual to move within that structure responsibly and to his own benefit. This awareness of the true nature of freedom will grow as we become more aware of the structure and order within which we ourselves live and of the enormous freedom that that structure does in fact give us.

With such a change in approach, no longer will we be able to see a classroom of 20 to 40 children as simply 'another group of little pests who have to be got through another day'. Each class will be seen as a collection of totally unique individuals, each with the possibility of becoming, by our current standards, a genius in one field or another. With such an approach the current shackles that we place on young human beings will finally begin to fall away.

In addition to these points, major changes will be made in the information taught to children. Rather than trying to inculcate them with facts from various disciplines that we consider important, children will be given basic information about how they function, with guidelines for directing them to special areas of interest and importance. Subject matter will also change as we increasingly realise that the retentive power of the brain means that everything we 'put in' will stay in, and will eventually—in either a clear or disguised form—come back.

Education will also expand its current boundaries, continuing throughout lifetime, and shedding its current emphasis on age. Our current and false assumptions about the decline of mental facility with age are already beginning to crumble. As this new realisation becomes an increasing part of general consciousness, whole areas of social change will be brought about. Rather than condemning our 'aged' to lives of useless isolation and decline, the great resources of their combined experience and memory will be put to use in a new mobile area for the benefit of society as a whole. This will include an education system which will allow individuals to co-operate, congregate and learn as a function of interest and level of knowledge, rather than as a function of age grouping.

Our knowledge of words and symbols, and the way in which they interact in our minds, will also have deep-rooted effect on our future social interactions and education systems. The fact that each word has millions of possible hooks, and that each individual will have a different series of combinations of associations for each word, means that we have no choice but to accept a more flexible and understanding approach to communication than we have hitherto done. As this flexibility, relativity and individuality in communication increases, it is possible that many of the arguments currently brought about by rigidity of definition, and by 'identifying by -isms' will subside.

The new nature of our understanding of words will also change the way in which we use them. Rather than forcing them into only sentence and linear structure, we will become far more flexible, creative and relevant in our use of them. As shown in Chapter 2, work in this field has already indicated that by using words for recall and creativity in conjunction with new knowledge about how the brain works, recall can be improved from an average of 40% to an average of 95%, and creativity can be increased by *tens* of times.

All this information begins to sound a little like the predictions of the future possibilities of man outlined in past science fiction novels. Not surprisingly, much of science fiction becomes science fact, and it now seems more probable than it did in the past that many of mankind's continuing dreams about his own potential may be on the verge of becoming true. The age-old dream of controlling matter with the mind is already true as far as the human system is concerned. Many people in different countries around the world can already control functions which were previously thought to be beyond their control: heart rate can now be adjusted at will, temperature can be raised and lowered; pain can be suppressed; metabolic levels can be adjusted at command; and brainwaves can be 'played' like the tunes of a musical instrument.

The recurring dream of perfect memory is not only now theoretically possible, but in fact has been achieved by the Russian 'S'. The pinacle that 'S' reached no longer seems so impossible when recent research shows that by the development of our individual sense-awareness, and by development of specific techniques and approaches to the art of memory, extraordinarily accurate recall can be attained by 'the average man'. Other science fiction ideas also seem to be closer to realisation. The concept of perfect mimicking seems more possible in view of our new understanding of the mind's ability to control muscles. Extraordinary control of groups of muscles has been achieved by a number of individuals, the process being likened to a perfect puppeteer, in which the mind pulls the infinite number of strings required to change the physical appearance of the face. Similarly, in imitation of the voice, individuals who could control the resonance of the intricate series of caverns and chambers in their cranium have reproduced sounds with incredible accuracy.

Other science fiction concepts, such as the transfer of the body from place to place by identification-through-memory and the ability to see in the future, although far from realisable, are already being given 'serious concern' by recognised institutions. Our awareness of the expanding universes within our mind has coincided with the awareness of the increasing relative smallness of our own planet in the universe, as Edgar Mitchell, the sixth man to walk on the moon, pointed out in Chapter 5.

Our increasing awareness of our true place in the universe, of our own true potential, and the increasing sophistication of our mechanical service systems, brings the concept of a world brain closer to realisation. Already, like the individual neurons within the brain, each of us is becoming increasingly independent, and increasingly interdependent. As long as this can be linked with an ever-increasing self-awareness—and an ever-increasing sense of social responsibility will be inevitable—it even seems possible that the utopian dreams of the visionaries of the past may well be in sight.

As we increasingly delve into what is becoming known as the 'mind-mine' it appears more and more that we are entering a new renaissance. It even appears that this new renaissance may be able to produce, as a result of our increasing knowledge of ourselves, the new renaissance man. No longer will the charge be viable that the 'complete man' is impossible because the mind cannot take in all the information available. With the new broadening of the mind the possibility now exists that once again we can embrace the sciences and the arts as well as nurturing the physical and spiritual aspects of our existence. The new renaissance man will be a super version of that envisioned in the fifteenth century.

Like the other areas of human endeavour at the present time, the area of the mind is still unresolved, and still involved in turmoils as different institutions and different cultures propose their own theories, explanations, and suggested functions for man's mind. This turmoil, like the turmoil in other areas, can be seen more happily when compared to converging rivers. Where a number of large rivers converge, there will inevitably be massive turbulence. It is the same with different cultures and different ideas: when they initially come together there is a period of violent disagreement and disruption, giving the impression of confusion and chaos. Shortly after the junction of the meeting of rivers, a larger, smoother and calmer river flows. Again it will hopefully be the same with the coming together of our different cultures and different minds.

From within this apparent turmoil, we may well be forging the next leap in evolution—the advancement of our minds through a more enlightened individual and group consciousness.

10 Summary and Projection

Present knowledge; a fantasia of the future; a developing awareness
A personal view by Tony Buzan

The universe began twenty billion years ago. Mankind's planet, earth, has existed for only a fraction of that time. Man himself has existed on his earth for only a fraction of *its* billions of years. For those two million years that he has existed, he has been civilised for only a very few thousand. It took him most of those few thousand years to find out where his brain was located, for even by the time of the Greeks, most philosophers and scientists assumed that the brain was a function of air and water currents, and even Aristotle assumed that most of the functions we now attribute to the brain were located in the heart. It is only in the past few hundred years that man has known where the seat of his consciousness was located. And it is only within the last few decades that the bulk of his knowledge about himself and his mental processes has been gathered.

Against this background of the millenia, our new explosion in self-knowledge can be seen as the seed that it really is. From it may grow a future that will truly amaze.

Left and right
The work of Robert Ornstein (see Chapter 6) on the hemispheres of the brain has already shattered many of our cherished and unworthy assumptions about our individual capabilities. The fact that one side of our brain controls logic, mathematics, analysis and language, while the other controls rhythm, music, imagery, imagination and spatial relationships, brings into question the labelling of people in the past as either scientific or artistic, either left-hemisphere or right-

hemisphere biased. Very often in the case of those labelled artistic, they not only suffer the disadvantage of the withering of the scientific side, but also the added stigma of being considered somehow less intelligent, because the society of the time arbitrarily places 'higher' values on one form of mental activity than another.

Ornstein's discoveries not only lay such historic assumptions conveniently to rest, they also emphasise that within each person lies the possibility of both the scientist *and* the artist. Such a blending of potentials has already shown benefits, individuals having shown increments of improvement not in fractions but in entire units because of the stepladdering effect when one side of the brain stimulates the other, establishing a positive spiral of reinforcement. (See Chapters 2 and 3.)

Ornstein's work has also raised our general level of self-awareness, and the future benefits may very well be incalculable. Apart from significant increases in artistic activity in societies which have been science-oriented, and scientific activity in societies which have been artistically oriented, further specific advantages will additionally accrue with this increased awareness of the individual range of aptitude and 'mentalities'

It may seem absurd to suggest that much precious information has been deliberately thrown away by people in the past, yet it may not be so far from the truth. Many people report having dreams in which, at the time, they think they have come up with world-shattering revelations which they dutifully note on their bedside scribble-pads. Upon reading their scribbled notes when awake, they find such 'ridiculous' statements as 'the solution to the universe is a banana'!

Before throwing away any such 'message' you might write to yourself in the future, it may be useful to bear in mind the fact that such messages may well come from the right hemisphere of the brain, which does not operate on the same conceptual level as the brain's left hemisphere. When waking we immediately switch into 'conscious' mode, which tends to be a left-hemisphere dominated form of activity. Thus we look at our right-hemisphere message with our more verbally logical left-hemisphere, and reject what we read as absurd. This may be an error, a misreading, for very often the imagistic/conceptual side of the brain formulates its solutions in

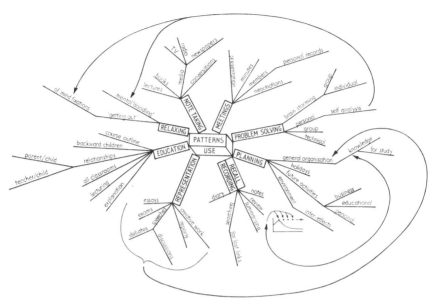

Brain patterns and their uses

Astonishingly, this 1930's advertisement is selling 'modern science'; our perception today would be somewhat different

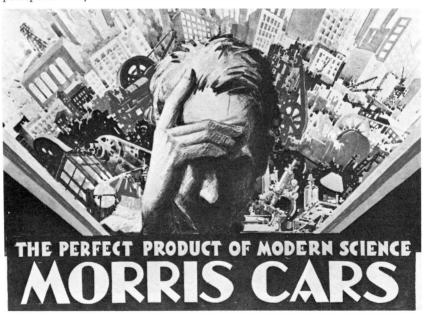

THE PERFECT PRODUCT OF MODERN SCIENCE
MORRIS CARS

parables. Thus, if the dreamer of the banana parable had been an Albert Einstein, he might have been able to unearth the clue 'curved'.

Up and down

In addition to our left-right polarity, we also have an up-down polarity, the difference between the cortical layers which house our more complex intellectual functions, as well as the discriminating processes, and the 'lower' or thalamic regions—often known as the 'old brain'—which house our 'basic' emotions. Our understanding of the inter-relatedness of these functions is already having an impact on all levels of society, and will continue, increasingly, to do so.

We already know that when the cortical and thalamic regions are not integrated, mental functions become disintegrated. The behaviour noticed in such instances is described as over-emotional, neurotic, or even mentally ill. What is often happening is that parts of the brain are rebelling against other parts; the brain is becoming fragmented and divided against itself, often setting up vicious circles in which an emotion such as fear from the thalamus stimulates the rest of the body and other nerve-centres, which themselves send messages back to the thalamus, which then sends out *more* fear-messages, leaving the person in states which can range from general tension, through helplessness to, in extreme cases, complete unconsciousness.

Integration of these two levels would hopefully bring about not the oft-parodied 'cold' individual, but one sensitively balanced, whose cortical and discriminative capabilities would savour the infinite emotional themes and differences of the emotional strata, 'interfering' only when the emotion became such as to damage the individual, other individuals, or the environment. With such cortico-thalamic control, much distress and shock can be withstood, much illness averted, and much unnecessary stress avoided.

Although we are only at the beginning of this balancing awareness, already major breakthroughs have been made in the related areas of biofeedback, meditation, self-hypnosis and auto-suggestion. We now know that it is possible to control with our cortex blood pressure, temperature, circulation, heart-beat, digestion and pain centres. From the personal stories of athletes and people in physical emergencies, we know that it is possible to produce imagistic 'sets' that enable the body to direct what were previously thought of as super-human emotional forces against apparently insurmountable physical odds, and to succeed. And we further know that this self-control can extend, in certain instances, to life and death. There are numerous medical and cultural reports of people 'who should have died' but who, by some 'superhuman act of will' managed to survive the impossible.

Our self-will can also be used to bring about death. This often happens when the individual feels there is nothing left to live for, as in the case of the loss of a dearly loved spouse, relation, or role. There are many instances where, when one partner has died, the other has 'set' him or herself to die *within hours*. Similarly, the aborigines in Australia can set themselves to stop living if they and their society feel that death is warranted. In such situations no amount of traditional medical interference can change the course of events upon which the aboriginal mind has set itself.

We now know that such self-control *can* be effected, and we now know more about *how* it can be effected.

The future will probably see a much greater general development of cortical-thalamic integration, and it is not unreal to expect that individuals will be able to combine the various aspects of meditation in which we currently indulge, adding to them with new knowledge, to produce combined meditations that will be more successful than those of the current day, and which might well sound like this to the mind's inner ear:

> drift from active-consciousness . . . float to other levels . . . free the energy meridians . . . open awarenesses . . . allow the aortal flow . . . dilate all capillary filaments . . . establish flow-perman-ence . . . listen to the body's many sounds . . . enter the complete mini-hibernation . . . establish and allow-to-be-satisfied the cell-needs . . .

The commercial image of biofeedback (*Aleph One Ltd, Cambridge*)

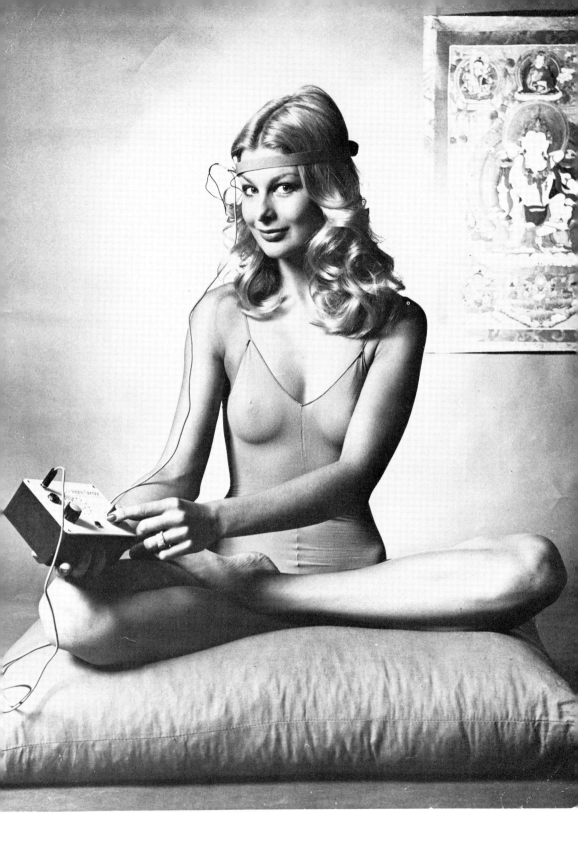

Brain cells

Pyotr Anokhin's foundation-shuddering revelation that

> ... we must consider the individual neuron and the millions like it as a system possessing innumerable degrees of freedom established in the brain by the multilateral synaptic connections between neurons. Simple mathematical calculation shows that the number of 'degrees of freedom' throughout the brain is so great that writing it would take a line of figures, in normal manuscript characters, more than 10·5 million kilometers in length! With such a number of possibilities, the brain is a keyboard on which hundreds of millions of different melodies— acts of behaviour or intelligence—can be played ...

has also changed the way in which we see ourselves.

Knowing that each of our ten billion individual brain cells has ten million, million, million, *million* degrees of freedom, and that each of these brain cells is both independent and interdependent, we can draw no other conclusion but that each individual's potential is much greater than had been hitherto thought (see Chapter 4), and that each individual is far *more* individual. A comparison between brain cells and the brain, and individuals and society, is a tempting one: just as the brain cannot function without its individual cells, and just as the cells cannot function without their brain, so it is with man and society; and just as each brain cell is intricately and intimately linked with its main body, so is each human individual with his society. The pendulum-swinging of the past in discussions about the relative importance of the individual versus the society may well come to a convenient rest with the realisation that such discriminations are not intrinsic, that each is interdependent with the other, and that to separate either, conceptually or actually, destroys both.

The delicately interwoven and fantastically interlaced network that is our brain gently vibrates and hums with a multitude of brainwaves—ethereal transmissions of which our relatively clumsy measuring instruments have managed to pick up at the moment only five: the Delta waves when we sleep; the Theta waves which indicate 'moodiness'; the Alpha waves which indicate our meditational states; the Beta waves which indicate our active states; and the waves which indicate the 'field' around nerve fibres as messages pass from one to another. Our technological sophistication in this area has been compared to someone who, wishing to monitor simultaneously every conversation in a large metropolis, holds an ordinary microphone two miles above the centre of the city, and interprets the general noise that he records as the 'absolute truth'.

In the future we will doubtless encounter many other forms of waves, more subtle even than those we now measure, and with a greater understanding of this aspect will come an even greater self-awareness and self-control. Even now many people are able to produce, at will, any of the Delta, Beta, Alpha and Theta waves for the improvement of their general mental wellbeing.

Holography

The most sophisticated piece of technology yet applied as a metaphor for the functioning of our brain is the laser-produced, laser-decoded, three-dimensional photograph or hologram. The hologram reproduces a three-dimensional image, which hangs in space, and which can be walked around to reveal its different aspects. The photographic plate on which the holographic image is stored can be shattered into hundreds of pieces, yet each piece will still retain the entire image. Many psychologists and brain researchers still consider the holograph to be the 'last word' as a model for the brain functions, suggesting that perception, cognition, retention and recall can all be explained by the use of this model. As so often happens with last words, however, they can simply signal the beginning of an entirely new set of even more complex questions. So it is with the brain.

To get a glimpse of this complexity, close your eyes and imagine an ideal little daydream-story in which you have characters, settings and events, and which is preferably in colour. Give the events some form of plot, and if possible attempt to 'see' the various physical aspects and angles of the settings and characters. Once you have done this, and if you still feel that the holograph is an adequate explanation for total brain function, answer the following questions:

Where did the colours come from?
Who and what moved the holographic images?
How were they moved?

Where did the props come from?

Where were the characters filed?

Who or what invented the plot?

How many other plots, characters, sets, props, changes, and angles could have been imagined; if nearly limitless, where would *they* come from?

and finally, and perhaps most important of all:

Who was watching the show?!

It is the answer to these questions which will provide one of the next major breakthroughs in our understanding of our own brains. And it is similarly the answers to these questions which will provide an even greater array of consequent questions . . .

Special instances of brain aptitude

Recently, increasing information has been coming to light about individuals who, apparently no different from anyone else, developed by chance abilities which may probably lie dormant in most of us. In many of these instances the individuals considered themselves normal, and were surprised when others considered them to be in any way different. This common assumption on their part, when considered in the light of Anokhin's statements about the enormous uniqueness of each individual, augurs well for the future, for it suggests that there are probably millions of individuals considering themselves normal 'like everyone else' when in fact they are normal with specially developed abilities in certain areas.

Among those special cases recently come to light is that of the visual researcher, W. H. Bates, who when investigating the extent of normal vision, discovered a young girl who claimed that she could see the moons of the planet Jupiter. It was considered impossible with the unaided eye, but was checked by asking her in what position with relation to the planet she saw them. Her description of their location coincided identically with information provided by astronomers.

The Russian 'S' who was studied by Pyotr Anokhin's student, Alexander Luria, had developed a virtually perfect memory from the time of his childhood. He was able to memorise everything that Luria asked him to, sometimes recalling in perfect detail, complicated tests that he had been given twelve years earlier! 'S' also reported that his perfect memory was somehow associated with the fact that all his senses combined on every image his mind formed; he smelt, saw, tasted, felt and heard *everything*. His natural gift is one that can be partially duplicated by the learning of special memory systems called mnemonics, which not surprisingly rely for their success on an extensive use of the right hemisphere of the brain, especially its ability to imagine and exaggerate. His memory capabilities are more common than might be thought—many children are able to 'photograph' scenes and are able to read them back at a later date in almost perfect detail. This ability, again related to the right hemisphere of the brain, is often 'trained out'. There is no reason why, with proper training and retraining, each individual could not develop a memory many times more effective than it is at present, ranging from specific details such as numbers, names and faces, etc through to 'whole scenes' which could be registered in a mnemonic blink.

Pieter van Jaarsveld, a South African boy, became famous at the age of 12 in 1963 because of his 'X-ray eyes' which could detect water deep underground. Unlike other water diviners, he used no dousing rods, but said that he was able to see water 'shimmering like green moonlight' underneath the ground. This ability, which at first seems astounding, is rendered less so when it is considered that the brain itself is composed of 65% water, and to assume that its high state of consciousness could *not* detect the waves of its own element might be perhaps more surprising.

People with multiple personalities are often considered 'freaks' or mentally disturbed, but when looked at in the light of the brain, no matter what else one labels them, they are human beings who are able to house in one brain more than three 'individuals'. This ability, perhaps most famous in the case known as the three faces of Eve, is virtually absolute: every psychological test on each of the personalities confirms that they are definitely different and that each personality is complete and internally consistent. This ability to 'identify' on many levels, if unshackled from the bonds of fear in which it is often bound, could have untold advantages in terms of human understanding and interrelationships, not to mention acting!

Rosa Kuleshova is a Russian woman who, though not blind herself, grew up with a family of blind people whom she helped by learning to read braille. She taught herself to do other things with her hands, and in 1962 her physician took her to Moscow where the Soviet Academy of Science confirmed that she could see with her fingers. Under test conditions it was established that she could, with her hands, differentiate the three primary colours, that she could read newsprint and sheet music under glass and could distinguish the colour and shape of patches of light projected onto her palm or shown on an oscilloscope screen. After the announcement of her genuineness, the Russians did follow-up studies, and found that at least one in six people was able, after training of short duration, to learn to recognise the difference between at least two colours, and that this could be done not only with the hands, but also with the elbow and other parts of the body.

As with the information on other aspects of the brain, these case studies are now 'known'. The possible message they bring is not that there are a few freaks who stand out above the rest, but that latent within each individual lies the possibility for a level of consciousness that had previously been thought only available in characters from fiction.

The information that enters the brain

It has long been an established law of western philosophy that 'identicals' are 'different'. For example, two chairs from the same set, though looking alike at first glance, when examined in detail—down to the finest molecular level—are different in thousands of millions of ways. In view of what we have recently discovered about the human brain, this law can now be seen to apply especially to the human situation; each brain, although generally 'like' others, is specifically different not only in millions but *billions* of ways.

This law applies also to the information which each brain receives. Every word, every number, every image, every symbol, is not an absolute, but is relative—a multi-ordinal or many-hooked centre from which can radiate an almost infinite number of different meanings. Every word that an individual uses differs in its meaning-associations from every other word that the individual uses and, more important-ly, every word used by an individual differs in its meaning-association from the *same* word used by every other individual. Our words and symbols are abstractions from reality, and as such are merely shadows or imperfect mirrors of that which we would describe. Our

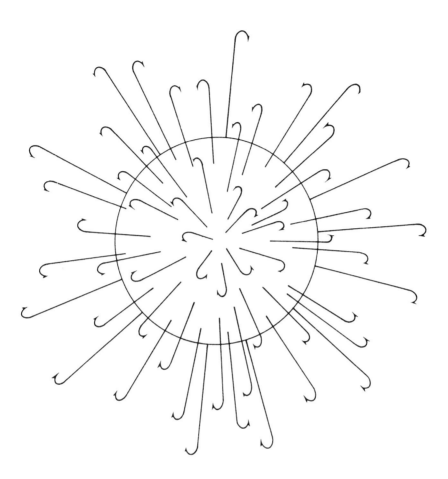

Every word, every number, every image, every symbol, is not an absolute, but is relative – a multi-ordinal or many-hooked centre from which can radiate an almost infinite number of different meanings

descriptions, of necessity, hint at only a few of the more generalised qualities of that which we would convey.

In the brain of each human there exists a vast multi-million-centred network of relative meaning-nodes, linked to each other by associations that have been built up by the individual throughout his or her lifetime; by associations that are uniquely personal.

This relative/associative breakthrough in our understanding of the information that feeds our minds explains how the associations around the word 'fish' were so different among the nine-year-old non-University children described in Chapter 2. These extraordinary and unique differences exist for all words in all minds, and apply just as much to 'fish' as they do to words like 'capitalist', 'communist', and 'God'.

This new knowledge on how the vast and intricate individual brain meshes and interweaves with the equally intricate world of information opens the way for improvements in many areas of human functioning. It helps us, for example, to understand more clearly the nature of understanding and misunderstanding. In this new light understanding can be seen as the sum total, up to a given time, of a person's information intake, and the links that have been made between the various elements of that information. Misunderstanding between individuals is often based on a false assumption made by one or both of them that the symbols and words they use are somehow absolute and unchanging. Altercations often arise not because there is necessarily fundamental disagreement, but because the words being used have different associations for each of the individuals. In the modern world this is increasingly a problem between epistemic communities, where the translated simile conceals meanings which are often in direct opposition. The sooner this knowledge about our brains and the information they receive is disseminated, the sooner will such faulty disagreements be registered as symptoms of our 'uneducated past'.

The knowledge about the associative nature of the brains and the information they receive is also beginning to liberate us from the linear tyranny in which formal grammar has placed us for the last few hundred years. Standard grammar and formal sentence structure are, and probably will remain, one of our main forms of inter-communication. They are not, however, the only forms, and the expansion of our flexibility in the use of words is already demonstrating itself in the use of 'brain patterns' for such tasks as creative thinking, problem solving, brain storming, note taking, speech making, planning, general communication and education. Using symbols and language in this brain-related way has already produced improvements which are as significant to mental performance as was the use of the engine to transportation.

Education

Education has progressed from the times of the dark ages, when very little was taught, to a stage where it can now select and present an astoundingly wide variety of information that we hope will be useful to those we teach. As a consequence, our colleges of education teach our teachers to teach facts. For a number of years this process proceeded satisfactorily, but in the last decades a new bottleneck is being experienced: there is too much information to teach, and both teachers and students are being swamped.

This current dilemma can be eased by changing emphasis. Instead of teaching teachers to teach facts, we must now teach teachers to teach students how to learn. Rather than teaching about history, religion, language, mathematics, physics and so on, we must teach children at very early stages about their basic mental and learning functions: how their recall works during the learning period; how iheir eyes move when they read; how they can vary the speed of tntake of their information; how to organise thought; how to solve problems; how to think creatively; how to review successfully; how to make adequate notes in brain pattern form; in all, how to study in a flexible way that will make the whole process of learning an enjoyable and exciting one, rather than the comparatively boring tedium which it has become for so many people.

And at the very beginning of the process we must inculcate children with the trust that they *can* learn. Our brains are so sensitive, and so delicately balanced, that often one word or phrase in a positive or negative direction can change a person's self-image for the rest of his life. In a recent survey of English Universities and Businesses, it was found that *more than 50%* of people questioned were convinced that they were almost completely incompetent in either art or mathematics. When pressed for proof of the fact, they invariably reverted to a statement by an early teacher who had told them so. Having once been 'programmed' to this 'knowledge' they acted on it for the rest of their lives. Ornstein's work on the left and right hemispheres of the brain, showing that each person has a considerable potential in both areas, is the first large nail in the coffin of this educational prejudice.

Once a child has been taught to learn, using even only a fraction more of his brain's potential, he will be able to range far more freely and easily over the fields of knowledge, comfortably accelerating the process by a factor of five to ten times the current rate. Such a factor may seem alarmingly significant, but it seems less so when it is considered that even our most able students at the moment have forgotten 80% of what they learnt in formal education within three months of graduation.

In conjunction with this new approach to teaching children how to learn, and of teaching them that each experience contains its lesson, a new approach will have to be taken toward testing. We now test a situation which we have in fact created ourselves, and then measure what we mistakenly label 'basic potential' on the basis of the performance on our preconceived measuring grid. Children who have been taught, in the last few years, even some of the basic rudiments about using their brains, have already begun to make nonsense of some of the standard creativity, intelligence and general aptitude tests. Rather than being used as absolute measures of unchangeable ability, tests in the future will have to be used simply as measures of lack-of-training, low scores reflecting not entirely on the person who makes the score, but also on the teachers who had as yet been unable to help the child past that particular learning stage.

The education of the future will also have to include an untangling of the concepts of order and rigidity, and freedom and chaos. We have often confused order with rigidity, and freedom with chaos. Rather than having classrooms specifically regimented in terms of subject matter and time, or classrooms in which everything is random in order to foster 'creativity', classrooms will combine a basic organizational structure with a freedom for the individual to move within that structure responsibly and to his own benefit. This awareness of the true nature of freedom will grow as we become more aware of the structure and order within which we ourselves live and of the enormous freedom that that structure can in fact give to us.

Education will also expand its current boundaries, continuing throughout lifetime, and shedding its current emphasis on age. Our current and false assumptions about the decline of mental facilities with age are already beginning to crumble, especially under the weight of information such as that of Rosenzweig, whose work has shown that the human brain, rather than becoming rigid, can develop an increasing plasticity as it goes through life. As this new realisation becomes an increasing part of general consciousness, more areas of social change will be brought about. Rather than condemning our 'aged' to lives of useless isolation and decline, the great resources of their combined experience and memory could be put to use in a new mobile area for the benefit of society as a whole. This will include an education system which will allow individuals to cooperate, congregate and learn as a function of interest and level of knowledge, rather than as a function of age grouping. Perhaps, as in previous and other societies, the aim of education will not be to produce people who are 'burnt out' and 'over-the-hill' by the age of 40, but to produce people who warrant such titles as 'Elder' and 'Sage'.

Such an educational system would hopefully produce well rounded and well balanced individuals, who still retained the innocence and inquiring nature of childhood, combined with widely accumulated knowledge and wisdom of experience. The nature/nurture argument, which sets the basic aptitude of the individual against the effects of education and environment, will also be laid to rest beside arguments such as the individual/group argument. We are now beginning to realise that the nature of the human brain is almost unbelievably rich and potentially harmonious. It obviously needs the most nourishing, favourable and loving nurture in order to flourish.

A fantasia of the future

Oysters removed from their original seabed and carried a thousand miles away, there being placed in light-sealed containers, adjust themselves with perfect accuracy to the earthly and universal rhythms which they are still able to detect. A seaweed 'knows' the position of the moon in the sky. A moth, thirty miles from a potential mate, can detect one molecule of her smell among billions. The mature salmon and eel can navigate their way through thousands of miles of shifting waters to find *exactly* the place at which they were spawned. Monarch butterflies travel thousands of miles from all regions of the northern hemisphere to congregate in an area a few hundred yards wide in Central America. The snowdrop can detect, with unerring accuracy, the rhythms of activity on the surface of our sun.

With the knowledge that plants and creatures from such early stages of our evolutionary tree have such fantastic and subtle abilities,

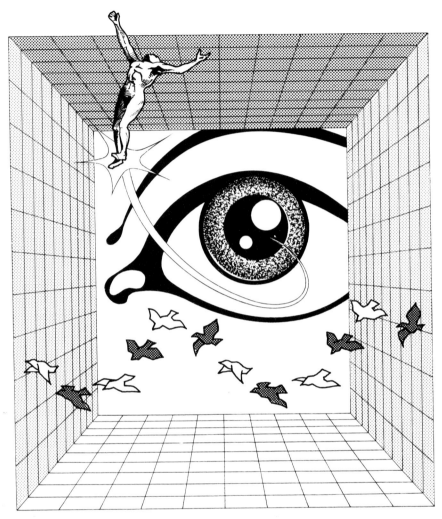

and with the recent knowledge of the enormous sophistication of the human organism, often described as the flower of the evolutionary tree, can we justifiably give ourselves limits?

Let us suppose not, and explore the possibilities.

Development of the senses

If you take all the 'space' from between the molecular structures that make up a human being, condensing him into solid matter, that solid matter would be a speck no larger than the size of a pinhead. We are, in the real sense, tiny specks of matter strung together by gigantic energy wave sources, and we communicate and survive by exchanging our vibrations with those of the universe. Using our gigantic brains as the overseers and directors of this energy force, there is no reason to assume that we cannot develop our senses to extremes previously considered impossible. In the future we may be able to see what now can only be seen with the microscope and telescope, naturally taking in the landscapes of the macro- and micro-cosmic. Using our eyes, and perhaps more than our eyes, we may be able to discover new colours in the spectrum, to see the infra and ultra areas, and to perhaps detect even those waves which are so short that a few billion wave lengths cover less than a centimetre, and those waves which are so long that they travel through the universe in single strides of seven million miles.

And who is to say that we shall not be able to hear, taste, feel and smell as well as each of the multitudinous other life-forms that dwell with us on the planet? To listen to the sound of individual molecules tapping on the tympanum of our eardrum; to taste the different nuances in each particle of each solid and liquid that we take in; to detect in the air we breathe the multitudinous sensations of different smells and to feel, not just surfaces, but the vibrations from the molecular structures beneath them?

In this hyper-illumined sensory state, we may be able to truly observe ourselves, obtaining that dispassionate cognition which has for so long been the goal of man. Combining all senses into the hyper-illumined multisense, we may be able to observe the strands and filaments that make our very nature; to see the dancing molecular and atomic particles, to follow the spirals and linkages that compose the very nature of whatever it is that man is.

And with such power we might also be able to re-align the molecular structures within ourselves, directing many kinds of energies in many kinds of ways from any part of our body. In such a scenario, levitation, by directing energy against the weak force of gravity, becomes no longer a dream but a distinct possibility, as does creating matter from the energies from within and around us, simply by tapping, converting and moulding the energy from $E = MC^2$.

Prescience

If you were to take off from the earth, and travel faster than the speed of light, you would be able to look back at the light beams you had overtaken, and see yourself taking off, for perceived information travels only as fast as the light beam can carry it.

When you look up into the sky at night, everything you see is 'out-of-date' or from the past, some of it many millions of years old, having taken that length of time to travel the enormous distances between even the nearest stars in the universe and our own planet.

In a very real sense, the universe can be considered as a gigantic memory of itself, all events that have taken place being coded and carried somewhere on the Universal Wavelength Messenger Service. If this is the case, it is arguable that time, which we see as a fairly linear step-by-step progression, is in fact always 'now'.

If the past is being continually carried into the present, perhaps it is so with the future, and *all* time is now. If this is the case, then in order to 'tune in' to the future, all it requires is an instrument sensitive enough to gather and interpret the teaming and coded bits of information as they travel endlessly, and at the speed of light, around our speed-bound universe. Such an instrument may well be the brain.

In the future, or in the past, or now, we perhaps did, can, will, travel the corridors of time, as did Paul Atreides in Frank Herbert's *Dune:*

> Awareness flowed into that timeless stratum where he could view time, sensing the available paths, the winds of the future . . . the winds of the past: the one-eyed vision of the past, the one-eyed vision of the present and the one-eyed vision of the future— all combined in a trinocular vision that permitted him to see time-become-space.
>
> There was danger, he felt, of overrunning himself, and he had to hold on to his awareness of the present, sensing the blurred deflection of experience, the flowing moment, the continual solidification of that-which-is into the perpetual was.
>
> In grasping the present, he felt for the first time the massive steadiness of time's movement everywhere complicated by shifting currents, waves, surges and countersurges, like surf against rocky cliffs. It gave him a new understanding of his

prescience, and he saw the source of blind time, the source of error in it, with an immediate sensation of fear.

The prescience, he realised, was an illumination that incorporated the limits of what it revealed—at once a source of accuracy and meaningful error. A kind of Heisenberg indeterminacy intervened: the expenditure of energy that revealed what he saw, changed what he saw.

And what he saw was a time of nexus within this cave, a boiling of possibilities focused here, wherein the most minute action—the wink of an eye, a careless word, a misplaced grain of sand—moved a gigantic lever across the known universe. Abruptly, as though he had found a necessary key, Paul's mind climbed another notch in awareness. He felt himself clinging to this new level, clutching at a precarious hold and peering about. It was as though he existed within a globe with avenues radiating away in all directions . . . yet this only approximated the sensation.

He remembered once seeing a gauze kerchief blowing in the wind and now he sensed the future as though it twisted across some surface as undulant and impermanent as that of the windblown kerchief.

He saw people.

He felt the heat and cold of uncounted probabilities.

He knew names and places, experienced emotions without number, reviewed data of innumerable unexplored crannies. There was time to probe and test and taste, but no time to shape.

The thing was a spectrum of possibilities from the most remote past to the most remote future—from the most probable to the most improbable. He saw his own death in countless ways. He saw new planets, new cultures.

Matter transfer

It has been suggested in the annals of Sci-Fi that if two items could be attuned to a 20 decimal approximation of similarity, their molecules—unlike the molecules in the 'non-identical' philosophical chairs—becoming aligned similarly, the lesser of the two objects would be drawn to the greater much as magnet attracts magnet, and would bridge the gap in space, no matter what the distance.

This hypothesis becomes even more probable if time is all-present and if space is consequently a function of time. If time and space are in fact different manifestations of the same thing, then it is not unlikely that two objects which are truly identical would have to be in the 'same place'.

If the mind of Man could use the 'multisense' to 'super-perceive' any object, registering holographically the exact molecular structure, it might be possible for that human to instruct every cell to 'familiarise' the image of the desired object. If the object were larger than the man, the man would immediately be next to the object. If the object were smaller than the man, the object would immediately be next to the man, no matter what the 'distance' was originally between them.

Is it perhaps in such areas that future travel lies?

Alternatively, it may be possible to send out from an individual brain a 'bundle of consciousness' which could travel at the speed of light or faster around the universe, perceiving for the earthbound individual the realms of his cosmos, and either sending them back by wave, or returning them much as a cosmic reconnaissance scout.

And eventually Man might become the 'children of the universe', with an infinite playground in which to gambol, as imagined in this excerpt from the poem 'Structure in Hyperspace':

Their Toys! Their Fields!
Limitless limbs to drop rise kick hit and play!
Jewel clusters to glee over, spin, rotate; fireballs to form,
heat, condense rocks around, paint with gamut's brush, freeze,
explode; ball as sun, planet, molecule or atom to dribble, carry,
bowl, throw, kick, or spin, All to hurl, skip, swing,
rollick, clown, play pranks on, laugh, dally, romp through:
X-Ray gardens, gamma greenness, ultra, infra realities; Great
　　Wastes
Galactic clouds to peep from, blind man's buff in
Rorschach horses to mount and ride.

Around and around and through our straight circled speed
　　yoked universe!
riding on flame tailed iceballs, looking to rings looming
from Titan's only blue horizon, seeing filigree

of star-dust spectra tantalizing to us, laughing at: winged
    helmet;
slit symbolized; sphere crossed; war arrowed prick head; bolt;
Kronos; his spawner; trident; infernal god; and dust; our
    spinning stones;
kicking about blue stars full circling red as heat to blue is cold,
tampering with Cluster, Nebula, shackled suns, tandem
travellers, and Supergiant, absorbing all colours, seeing Monster
exploded into Crab, Light dust-belted, Supernova shattered,
and the Cosmos Red shift and Blue shifting us into cube
into cube into cube into nothingness in Everything.

Infinitely Energetic, Boundless, Unchained!

Telepathy and group mind

Using his electromagnetic wave-power, Man might be able to communicate with wave-tentacles directly and immediately with other
Man, and indeed with other creatures. In future he may be able to
pour his collected memory/identity from himself to another like
water into a chalice; to ride the intricate currents of the winds with
the mass-brain of a flock of birds; to see in the deepest areas of the
unknown ocean, reality through the millions of eye-brains of its
massed and moving inhabitants.

And eventually the mind may be the only instrument capable of
detecting the subtle changes in electromagnetic vibrations that
indicate the presence of life on other planets. If one impulse can
produce an electromagnetic field, then probably one race of beings
will produce a field also: a field which might effect minute and brain-
detectable changes in the universal matter around it.

Once these powers have been established, the possibility of the
group-mind or world-brain becomes a possibility, and Olaf Staple-
don, writing of the future in the early 1930s, will be realised:

> Very rarely and precariously has this supreme experience been
> achieved. In it the individual passes beyond his group experience,
> and becomes the mind of the race. At all times, of course, he can
> communicate 'telepathically' with other individuals anywhere
> upon the planet; and frequently the whole race 'listens in' while

157

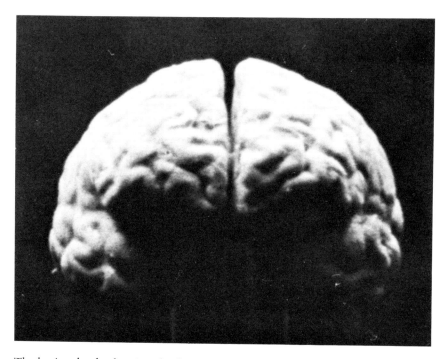

The brain, clearly showing the fissure separating the right and left hemispheres

one individual addresses the world. But in the true racial experience the situation is different. The system of radiation which embraces the whole planet, and includes the million million brains of the race, becomes the physical basis of a racial self. The individual discovers himself to be embodied in all the bodies of the race. He savours in a single intuition all bodily contacts, including the mutual embraces of all lovers. Through the myriad feet of all men and women he enfolds his world in a single grasp. He sees with all eyes, and comprehends in a single vision all visual fields. Thus he perceives at once and as a continuous, variegated sphere, the whole surface of the planet. But not only so. He now stands above the group-minds as they above the individuals. He regards them as a man may regard his own vital tissues, with mingled contempt, sympathy, reverence,

Gaseous Nebula in Gemini which by coincidence echoes the shape of the brain (*Hale Observatories*)

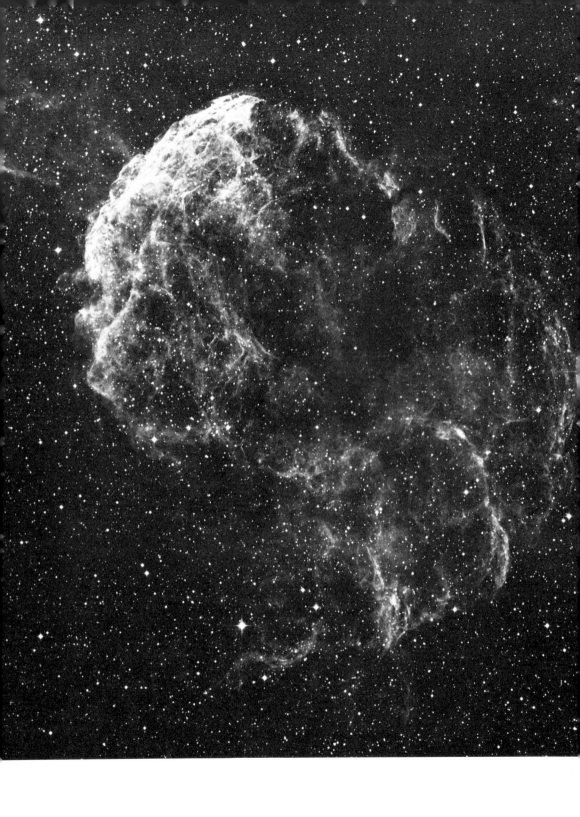

and dispassion. He watches them as one might study the living cells of his own brain; but also with the aloof interest of one observing an ant hill; and yet again as one enthralled by the strange and diverse ways of his fellow-men; and further as one who, from above the battle, watches himself and his comrades agonizing in some desperate venture; yet chiefly as the artist who has no thought but for his vision and its embodiment. In the racial mode a man apprehends all things astronomically. Through all eyes and all observatories, he beholds his voyaging world, and peers outward into space. Regarding the solar system simultaneously from both limbs of his world, he perceives the planets and the sun stereoscopically, as though in binocular vision. Further, his perceived 'now' embraces not a moment but a vast age. Thus, observing the galaxy from every point in succession along Neptune's wide orbit, and watching the nearer stars shift hither and thither, he actually perceives some of the constellations in three dimensions.

A developing awareness

At this present moment in earth's history, and for the first time in earth's history, *all* of earth's disparate civilisations and different mental streams are inexorably merging. The consequent confusion, fear, culture shock, and tendency to gloomy prediction is understandable, and can be lessened by looking at the major factors in the 'mix' and further looking ahead to the analogically prognosticated time of future calm.

In observing, Western Man has traditionally excluded himself from the event he was observing. Thus he assumed that he had no effect on the minute particles he weighed and measured, and also assumed that he had no effect on the living organisms whose 'objective' behaviour he tried to understand. He has carried this tendency to an extreme when considering the future of his societies, measuring and predicting only on the basis of sociological and psychological assumptions and generalisations, assuming that what is measured *is*, and not that what is measured can be changed.

Man's oversight in not measuring himself more accurately (a strange form of modesty!) has led him to conclusions that he would not have reached had he *had* more Knowledge. It is necessary, therefore, in order to gain a more complete understanding of our current situation, and a more probabilistic interpretation of our future, to look very closely at the main factor in all these discussions. This main factor is *not* the theories of economics or psychology, nor is it the 'basic aggressiveness of man' nor is it the 'irreversible tide of history'. The main factor, almost blindingly obvious, is that variable in the equation which is ubiquitous, which has been the subject of this book, and which in large part records, controls, and directs the rest of the equation: the human brain.

In our increasing understanding of this incredibly complex and mysterious organ, in our increasing understanding of ourselves and of our fellow men, and in our increasing understanding of the inter-connectedness and relativity of all things, lies the hope for the future.

In the ideally-envisioned future, mind will be in tune with body, mind with mind, and mind and body with the environment. The word 'selfish' will come to mean the same as the word 'altruistic', for anyone who is truly concerned with himself, being totally interlinked with everything around him, would be truly concerned for every-thing.

The divisive political systems of today will grow into bodies that will genuinely function for the good of all, and individuals within the society will be, by definition, totally interested in both the individual *and* the group, loving in the sense of desiring self-fulfilment for the beloved, with incidental self-fulfilment for the lover—each individual intimately and sensitively aware of the unique needs of him or herself and of the similarly unique needs of others.

Abstractions such as 'state' or 'nation' will no longer be exalted, for individuals will more realistically be aware of the true nature of our changing realities.

In such a state, conflict would arise not from an automatic fear and hatred of strangers, nor from a clash of wills based on half-truths considered as absolutes, but only from misunderstanding due to imperfect knowledge; misunderstandings which could be consider-ately and painstakingly worked out by exchange-of-information. In such a future world, mechanical computers will no longer be feared, and will have taken their appropriate place as assistants to the biological meta-and-super computers that gave them existence.

Languages, as they are beginning to do already, will blend into a single world language in which the subtleties, nuances, and number-less and unique cultural perceptions and informations will be shared by everyone.

In this new renaissance (for that is surely what it will be) medicine, communication, business and education will undergo gigantic changes for the better; a new polymath will arise, and he will be most people, educated to use his latent abilities to their full potential—no longer will the isolated envisionary have to live in deprived circum-stances suffering the rejection of others, but will be allowed to work in an atmosphere of social acceptance and encouragement; the fundamental principles of psychology, physics, art and chemistry, etc will probably be established as similar; and war between Man and Man will no longer exist. For Man is not warlike. His 'warlike' nature is based probably not on an innate desire to attack, but on an innate desire to preserve. Whenever he has been seen as violent, it is because he has 'truthfully-to-himself' defended the position he considered to be right. The only 'error' in this affection was that he assumed he had a complete knowledge of 'rightness' which in fact he had not at that time had the opportunity to receive. From the areas of both brain research and information theory, the nature of the relativity of that knowledge is now becoming apparent.

Such a utopia for mankind is only one of the vast array of fila-mental probabilities stretching into the future. Each filament can be swayed or broken by events as significant as the death of a world leader, or as apparently insignificant as 'the wink of an eye, a careless word, a misplaced grain of sand . . .'.

Looming behind these possibilities, and capable of exerting more influence on them than anything else, is the brain and mind of Man. With things as uncertain and as fluctuating as they are at the present time, it is essential that this enormous power be set towards realising the probabilities that will enable forthcoming generations to write magnificent future histories.

Bibliography

Bergamini, D. *The Universe* (Time-Life 1968)

Brierley, J. *The Thinking Machine* (Heinemann 1973)

Brown, P. (Ed) *Radical Psychology* (Tavistock Publications 1973)

Buzan, Tony *Speed Reading* (David & Charles 1977)

Buzan, Tony *Advanced Learning and Reading* (a manual)

Buzan, Tony *Use Your Head* (BBC Publications 1974)

Buzan, Tony *Speed Memory* (David & Charles 1977)

Clare, A. *Psychology and Dissent* (Tavistock Publications 1976)

Deaking, M. *The Children on the Hill* (Andre Deutsch 1972)

Doman, G. *Teach Your Baby to Read* (Jonathan Cape 1965)

Droscher, V. B. *The Magic of the Senses* (Panther 1971)

Firsoff, V. A. *Life, Mind and Galaxies* (Oliver & Boyd 1967)

Gooch, S. *Personality and Evolution* (Wildwood House 1973)

Heinlein, R. A. *Stranger in a Strange Land* (Berkeley Pub Corporation 1968)

Hess, H. *The Glass Bead Game* (Penguin Books 1973)

Huxley, A. *The Doors of Perception, and Heaven and Hell* (Penguin Books 1969)

James, W. *Psychology* (Fawcett 1963)

Julesz, B. *Foundation of Cylopean Perception* (University of Chicago Press 1971)

Klee, Paul *The Thinking Eye* (Lund Humphries 1961)

Lilly, J. C. *Centre of the Cyclone* (Paladin 1973)

Luria, A. R. *The Man with a Shattered World* (Jonathan Cape 1973)

Luria, A. R. *The Mind of a Mnemonist* (Jonathan Cape 1969)

Luria, A. R. *The Working Brain* (Allen Lane 1973)

Medawar, P. B. & J. S. *The Life Science* (Wildwood House 1977)

Newson, J. & E. *Patterns of Infant Care in an Urban Community* (Penguin Books 1965)

Ornstein, R. E. *The Psychology of Consciousness* (W. H. Freeman 1973)

Rapoport, A. *The Encyclopaedia of Ignorance* (Pergamon Press 1977)

Rapoport, A. *Human Aspects of Urban Form* (Pergamon Press 1977)

Russell, P. *The TM Technique* (Routledge & Kegan Paul 1976)

Sagan, Carl *The Cosmic Correction* (Hodder & Stoughton 1974)

Saint-Exupery, A. de *The Little Prince* (Heinemann 1945)

Skinner, B. F. *Beyond Freedom and Dignity* (Jonathan Cape 1972)

Steinhouse, D. *The Evolution of Intelligence* (Allen & Unwin 1974)

Suzuki, S. *Nurtured by Love* (Bosworth Press 1970)

Vogt, A. E. Van *The World of Null-A* (Sphere Books 1972)

Vogt, A. E. Van *The Pawns of Null-A* (Sphere Books 1974)

Watson, L. *Supernature* (Hodder & Stoughton 1974)

Watts, A. W. *The Way of Zen* (Pelican 1972)

Wilson, Colin *The Philosopher's Stone* (Panther 1974)

Readings from *Scientific American*, 'Perception Mechanisms and Models'

Readings from *Scientific American*, 'Altered States of Awareness'

Index

Page numbers in *italics* refer to illustrations